NINE LIVES

NINE LIVES

The Emotional Experience in General Practice

KENNETH SANDERS MD

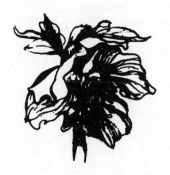

Clunie Press
for
The Roland Harris Trust Library
Monograph Series No. 5

Printed and bound in Great Britain by
Billing & Sons Ltd, Worcester

Contents

By the same author

A MATTER OF INTEREST : Clinical Notes of a psycho-analyst in general practice.

Acknowledgements

Once again, I gratefully acknowledge the debt to 'my friends pictured within.'

My thanks to Dr Philip Sanders for his interest, and for his help with proof reading.

My wife's participation has been indispensable at every stage and at all times.

Introduction

The transformation of an emotional experience into words is a worthwhile endeavor, but to do it in the form of a scientific paper seems to put it beyond the reach or interest of anyone except a few other specialists in the field.

The protagonists in the nine stories have all impressed their personalities on me in an unforgettable way. None of them would have wanted anything to do with psycho-analysis in its formal sense, and I cannot think why out of the melee of busy urban practice over nearly four decades, these nine lives, rather than any others, have come to be recorded in this way.

They have in common the fact that at their moment of need, I also had a need. I have tried to convey in these stories the nature of their vulnerability and sense of incompleteness. My neediness, the desire to respond and to record comes from the other side of the equation.

When, as a medical student, I first opened Samson Wright's Applied Physiology textbook, I discovered this epigraph inside,

> "Rabbi Akiba (in Roman captivity) to his favourite pupil Simeon ben Yochai: 'My son, more than the calf wishes to suck, does the cow yearn to suckle.'"

I had forgotten about it, until I re-opened the book after many years. I experienced the same sense of integration of cultures when, during the war years, a psycho-analyst was temporarily and mysteriously appointed to the staff of the psychiatry faculty, and for a term a refreshing zephyr of humanity suffused the arid lecture theatre. Then he disappeared back to London as mysteriously as he had arrived.

I subsequently learned during the course of my own analysis how extremely complicated, but how rewarding, the field of psycho-analysis can be, and in particular that the mystery of the connection between bodily illness and mental illness might not be explained, but could be studied. The technique for communicating this

1

activity, not surprisingly, turns out to be as problematical and difficult as the work itself.

Chapter One is the "scientific paper". "Nine Lives" is the same in story form. The Group Discussion of Chapter Eleven is a third version.

1   The emotional experience in general practice*

General practitioners have to think and act before all the information they need is available to them. No-where does this cause so much frustration as in emotional and psycho-somatic illness, where "information," in the sense of the basic sciences taught at medical school, is elusive, often incomprehensible, always controversial.

Psycho-analytic activity requires the courage and the imagination to permit a marriage between art and science. When they are separated, both remain sterile. In combination, they complement one another in an enhanced desire to find meaning in the experience of being alive.

Concepts of normal emotional development in children, also help to clarify the structure of disturbance, and thereby modify ways of thinking about many problem illnesses. But the psycho-analytic method which reveals those structures — comparable to the pictures of electron microscopy — is not easy to follow.

As with that instrument, and others at present in use in body-brain medicine, for example computerised tomography and other types of scanning, the pictures require experience to interpret. Most difficult of all for general practitioners trained in scientific method, is to accustom themselves to a shift in perspective to one which is mind orientated. This split between the idea of scientific and imaginative activity, between brain and mind, is from the psycho-analytic point of view, defensive about the pain of responsibility for inner reality.

What follows is an attempt to address the need and the desire of many general practitioners for some "hard facts" they can use, while enjoying the opportunity to deploy their intuitive sensitivity.

Freud, working with adults, described three structures in the mind: Id, Ego, and Super-Ego, the latter capable of improvement into an Ego-Ideal. In London, the presence of

* Contributed to the Third Workshop of Centro Studi e Ricerche in Medicina Generale, Turin, Italy. October 1989.

3

Melanie Klein from 1926 until her death in 1960 revived interest in child analysis. Children from the age of about two and a half, showed her that the mind was an inhabited world. This world of the imagination has always been known to the artist and poet. It is the stage in the theatre of Pirandello's mind where he discovered six characters in trouble, calling for help from an indifferent outside world.

The same Pirandello characters, mother, father and children caught the attention of Melanie Klein in the drawings and play of children. This family inhabits the mind, inhabits dream life, and profoundly affects perception of external reality. It is a picture that recalls Plato's cave, and has links with theological concepts of a holy family, outside and within. These connections with so many other human thoughts, the poetic imagination, the philosophical problem of epistemology, of what can be known about external reality and about ourselves, and the universal experience of religious feeling, led to a revival of interest in psychoanalysis.

The problem for the infant is to reconcile the parents in his or her mind with the real ones; the mother must attend to the discrepancy between the baby she has in mind, and the one of which she has been delivered. In the special case of a medical consultation, the doctor must compare the inhabitants of his or her mind, built up over the years of experience of being a child, a medical student, perhaps a parent, collate a conception of a healthy mind and body, and what is learned in studies of histology, pathology and bacteriology, compare this internal person with the present patient. The patient has the corresponding problem with the doctor.

Whenever two people come together, an emotional experience is possible. It may be welcomed as an opportunity for friendship or love; or the contrary, it may be feared, as a threat of intrusion. The prototype is the meeting of the baby with its mother and her breast and nipple.

In the psycho-analytic method, the analysis of the transference and counter-transference, analyst and analysand undertake to observe, report and think about the emotional experience of being with each other, with the aim of making contact with the original encounter with mother and father and siblings, and its possible unconscious interference with adult life.

4

Although freely entered into, there are times when the experience becomes unpleasant for both. There is conflict about getting acquainted with feelings. If sufficiently intense, they hurt.

The alternative is to evade the emotional experience, to hold the transaction at a commercial or even mechanical level. In medicine that happens when the patient is thought of as one machine that can be investigated by another. Both doctor and patient may fear the capacity to feel, while agreeing that it is a sign of life.

I want to compare analysis of the mind with investigation of the body. Unfortunately, they frequently become confused with one another. This is most noticeable at the time of conception: the idea that both mind and body have evolved from a fertilized ovum is so staggering that it is difficult to know what to think. It is a fact, like the existence of the universe, that is so perplexing that we agree, most of the time, not to bother about it. But between that moment of conception and the time forty years later when the ex-fertilized cell presents with a pain in its back, and asks for a diagnosis and cure, the distinction between a pain in the back and something that hurts at the back of its mind, is obscured by an almost impenetrable obstacle.

In a hospital, doctors learn to listen to the patient, examine the outer surface, then proceed to the inside. The body contains in its inner compartments amazing structures: heart, kidneys, intestines, lungs. There is that frightening substance, blood, of which we must be careful not to lose too much, not allow it to spill out of its container. There is the uterus, itself a container, in which, in common with so many animals, we have all had many months personal experience of being contained.

Work in the psycho-analytic consulting room gives access to the interior structures in the mind. If these structures deteriorate, like the great organs of the body, they begin to give rise to pain and anxiety. These "internal objects" are in psychic reality, internal parents and their children, and they inhabit the dream world, the imagination. They are felt to be distinct from the sense of self, and their pain is different. Most intriguing of all is the link between these internal structures in the mind, the internal organs of the body, and the experience of foetal dependence on the mother.

Toileting and feeding via the mother's kidneys and cardio-vascular system while the foetus is inside her, is taken over, when thrust into the outside world, by its own internal organs. But in its absolute dependence on maternal care it again participates in a process of mental and physical life being sustained by external and internal structures, over which it has no control. It is a very anxious situation. It is a model of the infant mind and body, externally dependent for its normal development on the body and mind of a family at work raising children, and the establishment of corresponding structures within itself.

Projective and Introjective Identification

From the start of life, a process of projection and introjection, is constantly at work. The baby takes the breast and nipple into its mouth, takes in the emotional experience of parental care. Over and over again, it loses some of what it has been given, throws it back into the external world at the other end of the gastro-intestinal tract. Thus also with emotional incontinence: gratitude and satisfaction for maternal care alternate with out-bursts of rage when frustrated. The infant gradually notices an important process: it is offered something valuable, at its head end, which keeps being evacuated at the bottom end. This is the paediatric heaven and hell, the Divine Comedy of life in the nursery.

This model of development has a further crucial step, the question of identification. The infant becomes confused about the real nature of the external parent, by these rapid fluctu-ations in its state of mind. If it has the experience of a good feed inside, it feels itself to be a good baby being looked after internally and externally by a good mother. If this alters to a smelly, faecal, internal parent, who can be defaecated out, it begins to suspect that the real mother or father also has deteriorated and instead of being friendly has become an enemy.

These fluctuations in the state of mind which confuse the infant about what is happening in its mind and body and the truth about the parents in external reality are difficult to describe, and extra-ordinary to experience, when, in an analytic session in adult life the same confusions can be demonstrated. For example, a young woman in the first week of her analysis, decribed her mother in the most contemptuous terms, but was also dissatisfied with her own identity as an adult woman. She claimed that her mother was only interested in her children if they were ill, not in their development. When I linked it with her fear that I was this bad mother to her baby self, she reported a dream in which the projection on an intrusive part of herself into the mother was clear: *"I was a spy in a peaceful village community. I wanted to leave, but in order to return to base, I had to avoid the police . . . . "*

In dream analysis, the detection by the analyst (*police*) of the secret intrusion by the infant self (*a spy*) into the internal parents mind and body (*peaceful village community*) may effect its withdrawal, with an improvement in the perception of the mother. This can be seen by the fact that the next day she referred to a letter from her mother, congratulating her on a promotion at work. As her own adult identity as a good mother, depends on the establishment in her mind of a good mother and father, the transition from super-ego, a bad parental object, to ego ideal, an admired one, is important.

Adult life according to this model is a secondary phenomenon. Feeling grown up, an insecure and variable experience, comes through identification, not with external parents – that might deteriorate into mere dressing up – but with internal parents. It implies that development proceeds only as far as imagination allows.

The family internally, is subject to the child's stormy passions, both of love and fury fuelled by frustration and jealousy, as in the external reality of family life. If things go badly the furniture may be broken. While the furniture of the mind may be shown in dreams as a house with chairs and tables, or a village in a landscape, these are symbols, the "poetic diction" of dream life, in which is embodied the values, the meaning of emotional life.

Sexuality remains a central issue in psycho-analysis. The focus of family life in both worlds is the sexual life of the parents, the mysterious and private world of adult lovemaking in which the children rightly assume they have their perplexing origin. The Oedipus complex relates not just to the murder of

7

one parent in order to marry the other, it may also contain an assault on the meaning of lovemaking, when adult sexuality is suspected to be not so much nutritious on the model of the nipple-in-mouth, but sado-masochistic and dirty minded like faeces-in-anus. In this way adult sexuality becomes confused with perverse infantile misconceptions.

The Protomental

If all goes well, the child's parents will help it to think about its experience of the external world, about which it receives messages from its sense organs. But it also receives sensations from inside, and not only from the body, but strange sensations, pressures, feelings, which if it could make sense of them might be recognized as emotional experiences. They are what have been called by Bion, "thoughts seeking a thinker".

The thinking is the mother's intuition about the baby's distress. She allows it to affect her, processes it in her own mind, and comforts the baby. This is maternal reverie. If internalized it will equip the baby to think for itself. This is a development in psycho-analysis — the concept of how learning from experience is possible. The idea is that the baby acquires the equipment from the parents.

If the mother's vitality is impaired, however, the infant may never receive the equipment in working order. From this point, Bion has developed the concept of the "protomental". The infant does not know what the pain he or she is suffering from is, whether it is the mind or in the body. Perhaps it is a pain that might develop into a depressive illness, a somatic one, a psychotic one, or even a psycho-somatic one. It is proto-mental: how can one differentiate wind from anxiety about when mother will come back? The problem persists, overlaid by the passing of the years, the maturing of the body. But it is still there, a difficulty in thinking about emotional pain. Twenty or forty years later, the patient may present to the general practitioner with a pain that defies explanation from a physical or chemical point of view.

The Reponsibility for Inner Reality: Persecution versus Depression

The concept of the infant receiving equipment from its experience at the breast, which furnishes the theatre of the mind with an internal family, leads to problems of responsibility for damage and loss. Methods useful in the external world: insurance, guarantees, return of damaged goods, legal disputes – none of these evasions are available. Depression about responsibilty for injury to the equipment, to the internal parents, may therefore change to a feeling of being threatened by them, as if they seek vengeance, like the ghost of Hamlet's father.

A theory of depression versus persecution was developed by Melanie Klein. Internal objects, like childhood toys have a short life. If all goes well, the infant learns to tolerate feelings of sadness about the repeated losing and re-gaining of its internal family and to learn from the experience to value his good objects, to struggle to protect them from harm and to use them and to identify with them: to develop an aesthetic sense of the beauty, sadness and mystery of the human condition.

When feelings of persecution are too powerful, well intentioned offers of help will not be welcomed as damaged internal parents become a focus of pathological identification to which access is denied. Anxiety about investigation of the interior of the mind may be compared with the history of the study of anatomy — the conflict between a thirst for knowledge, and mysterious inhibitions and fear concerning the inside of the body. Leonardo da Vinci and Versalius persisted and became heroes. It is something like that with Freud and Melanie Klein. It is something like that, in the work voluntarily undertaken by patient and doctor in partnership, on the investigation of what may be broken in the equipment in the of the mind.

Society has in general overcome its fears of the anatomical inside, although "the sight of blood" causes a tremor. With the mind, the problem persists. Treatment for the ill mind may be merely to stop it making a nuisance of itself, to "hit it with anti-depressants". The development of speech so useful for communication can also be used for disguising the truth about our selves. Our patients, like ourselves, hate to be thought "childish".

9

The Emotional Experience in General Practice

In general practice the opportunity to work in this field is boundless, and the need great, and while access to the inner structures of the mind is undeniably difficult, some familiarity with the available charts could be useful, for navigational purposes. The method, and the opportunity to transfer some of the mental pain from one mind to another, requires a readiness to allow oneself to be upset sufficiently to observe the pain, and bear the patient's suspicions. That is the toileting of distress.

But the doctor needs to be more than just a convenient receptacle for other people's pain and anguish. There is a desire to be nourishing, for creativity, to be active in the repair of something that is broken.

The removal of something unpleasant from the patient's mind and the gift of something good and valuable, that is not only relief from pain, but also the renewal of hope, may win thanks and even friendship. But the development of the mind, comes to an important threshold in childhood over this very problem of gratitude and friendship with their parents. Strong feelings of love and affection are painful, they bring with them an awareness of impermanence and loss, in a way that indifference avoids. The conflict is then seen to be not between love and hate, but between passionate, turbulent feelings which really hurt, and indifference which is pain free.

When patients work with the doctor in this way, they become puzzled, at the changefulness of their state of mind. They may leave feeling relieved of their distress, or angry and upset, or depressed and tearful, or indifferent. If one can help them to understand that love and hate are linked together, and that indifference is the problem, they may become curious, and want to know more, in conflict with the desire never to see you again.

The problem of hypochondria is present in medical practice at all levels, but it is the family doctor who is forced reluctantly to specialise in it. In psycho-analysis it has a precise definition: a pain in the mind that arises from identification with an internal object damaged in the conflict of passions roused by family life. The quality of the pain may be paranoid, persecutory: the patient feels sorry for him or herself, suspects that

10

the hospital has made a mistake, the pain is excruciating, and never leaves the mind in peace. Or, it may be depressive, a broken hearted lament for something, someone inside the mind or body that is failing, suffering, if only one knew how to reach them.

Strange indeed is the fact that when one takes an interest in hypochondria, it tends to retreat, to withdraw, at least in part and temporarily. The key to hypochondria depends on the reality of inner life. In the theatre of the mind, one of the characters has been struck down, is dead or dying or in pain. But it is not the self who is in pain, it is someone else, a parental couple has been attacked, the parents have been forcibly separated, they cry out for each other, the self feels responsible, identifies with the victim, feels the depressive or persecutory pain, is afraid of it and denies the reality of the life of the imagination.

If the doctor accepts a parental position in relation to the child in the patient, the crucial phenomenon of the transference will emerge. If the patient's internal family is in pain, the doctor will begin to feel the pain. If the patient is persecuted and blames others for the troubles, the doctor may observe a desire to protest in the tone of an irritated parent, "stop it, don't do that, I've had enough, go away and annoy some other doctor". If the problem is depressive, if the patient is feeling upset about a mistake that has caused some damage internally, then the response is more likely to be parental tenderness, and a desire to help someone so confused and dependent.

When I started practice in London in 1954, I was very puzzled by these problems. A few years later, embarked on an analysis, I began to think that the life of a psycho-analyst might suit me better. But I was surprised to find that I developed an interest in those very people who exasperated me so much.

One of them was a lady of about sixty, a housewife with a foreign accent whose husband, a timid dapper little man, whom I was treating for angina, died from coronary thrombosis. She was hypochondriacal, persistent, irritating, she looked and sounded terrible: stony eyed, blotchy complexion, wet nosed, a hoarse, expressionless voice, dressed in black in the outmoded fashion of the thirties. She had been investigated at hospital and there was nothing more to be done in that direction. She was hard to bear, she droned on monotonously, about the pain in her joints, her headache, her throat. It was impossible to re-assure her about her blood pressure, her bowels, her misery. If I spoke when she paused for breath, she looked at me sarcasti-cally, as if I was a street vendor, trying to sell her rotten vegetables, and we both knew it.

She was extremely adhesive, I was inexperienced. I didn't know how to insist that the consultation was at an end. She did not understand that when a doctor seizes his pen and writes the prescription, time is up. There was no way of ending the consul-tation other than by escorting her to the door and propelling her through it. She was obviously depressed, suffering from the loss of her husband, and pitiful in many ways. She aroused my anxiety, as well as my dislike. When she opened the door and I saw who was coming in, I felt my own blood pressure rise. After I pushed her out, I was slow to recover from the irritability that she had put into me, and I felt guilty that I had departed from my ideal of myself as a doctor.

But, in my analysis I found how good it was to have an analyst who could make contact with my inner life. One day I became curious about the effect of allowing this lady ample time to talk, and of trying to interest her in the new ideas I was learning. I invited her to come and talk to me when I had plenty of time, when I could listen, and of course think about what she told me.

She didn't come to the end of what she had to say in the first session. I had to push her out of the room at the end of an hour as I had at the end of fifteen minutes, but as I had been patient and generous with my time, I was at peace with myself. I invited her to come again a week later. She noticed the change in my behaviour, that I wasn't saying much other than questioning her a little about the events of her life. An improvement in the emotional atmosphere was perceptible. I was feeling more in control of my own consulting room, and she was feeling a little puzzled.

She submitted in the end to my method of conducting the interview and began to tell me about her life. It was eventful: she had come from Poland as a little girl and been brought up in a London that was almost Dickensian, at the turn of the century. After her mother's early death, she had helped her father, in his tailoring shop, in a small lane off Oxford Street.

When she met her husband, she helped him to set up a small draper's shop in Whitechapel, and raised two sons there. The business was successful, they moved to the suburbs, but it meant that her husband had a long journey to work every day on the Underground. If she had realised that he was going to have a heart attack, she would have insisted that he retire, they were not short of money, but he was the sort of man for whom work was his whole life. If only she had understood how ill he was, she would have been so much more careful to look after him . . . .

One of her sons was a comfort to her, he had qualified as a solicitor, and provided her with grandchildren. The other son was a problem, he had married a woman who didn't want children, who was jealous and possessive of her husband. There was to be a divorce, he was having an affair with another woman. Now that her husband had gone she lived alone in the house, it was too big for her to manage, a house where she felt her husband talked, telling her that she was not to blame . . . and so on. I had heard nothing of all this before, she wept while telling me about it, and I was moved, not only by her story, but by the transformation.

We went on like this for several weeks, until she commented on my behaviour, outside the bounds of her pre-conception of what a GP consultation should be. She may have thought that I was behaving like a psychiatrist – many people use that expression to denote their suspicion when one takes an interest in their lives – though I thought I was being psycho-analytic. She looked perplexed, quizzical, no longer sarcastic, but almost amused. I felt my identity had improved from a fraudulent street vendor, to a friendly milkman.

She couldn't make me out, I had made a move that had in some way outwitted her illness. We were having a kind of medical conversation but not much about aches and pains, more about the unique experience of the living of her life. I began to feel that she was in some way related to me, perhaps an eccentric aunt for whom I had become partly responsible.

Those moments when she started to notice me, first perplexed, later, after many months work, affectionately, were significant. It was as if she had not realised up to then that I was anybody in particular, just the doctor, of whom one can expect very little, certainly not that he would notice that *she* was anybody in particular. I have experienced the same thing since, in different patients, according to their personality and whether or not our work together went well. It is something that I have learned to look out for.

When the doctor complains that the patient is difficult, awkward, incomprehensible, when the patient gives pain, then a distressed internal object is projected into the mind of the doctor. The problem is to observe it, as a phenomenon, and think about it, while continuing to function in accordance with an ideal self; to observe the attempt to dislodge the identity of "doctor", for a character in the theatre of his or her mind. The element of reversal is characteristic when projective identification is operating: the patient makes the doctor feel worse, rather than him or her feeling better. If one can think about it, and not act on it, then the patient may be surprised to realize that in the theatre of the doctor's mind, the cast is different. There is then the possibility of identification with the ability to think. The patient's hitherto moribund internal parents and their family have the opportunity to revive. If this is accomplished, doctor and patient become important to one another.

Doctors are often advised to be careful of treating members of their own family because emotion gets in the way. But it is not unusual for a feeling of kinship to grow with the families in the practice. If a patient is ill or complaining, it might in a moment of confusion begin to seem as if they have materialized in this damaged state from a medical bad dream, and that the doctor is in some way responsible for the illness.

In fact of course, the doctor's responsibility in external reality is limited to making sure that he is not merely "such a good imitation of the real thing that it's impossible to tell the difference". But this in turn depends on an identification internally with good objects, who are permitted to carry out their maternal and paternal functions, without intrusion and control by disconsolate child parts of the self anxious to dress up and play at doctors and nurses.

In summary, I have drawn on the psycho-analytic blossoming of recent decades, associated with the work of Freud, Klein and Bion, to describe an approach to the human problems met by all family doctors. There is no "how-to-do it" manual in this non-mechanical matter, only learning from the emotional experience. Navigational guidance is offered for the use of those who are interested in this method of engaging imagination as well as hospital training in the art-science of general practice.

2   The spare man

Mrs Sadler lay, tremulous, on a sofa bed in the downstairs front room: in her late thirties, with an upturned nose, plucked eyebrows and hazel eyes, her prettiness was fading to mournfulness, her cheeks turning flat and pale, her hair straggly, mousy. She groaned, clutched her stomach, and frowned with pain.

She lived with her husband and three children in Grange Road, one of a cat's cradle of narrow streets, off Drapers Lane, a tributary of the High Street. The terraces were two up and two down houses, with front doors onto broken grubby pavements. There were no bathrooms, the outside toilets were through the kitchen door.

I was shown in by her husband, a Council labourer. He and his wife were uneasy with one another. She was pre-occupied with a vaporous jealousy, intermittently convinced that he was unfaithful. After a night of bickering, inflamed on both sides by bottles of Guinness, exhausted and benumbed by his plausible denials, terrified that she was mad and deluded, she had little energy for the morning, three children, and twenty minutes walk to her job in a factory canteen.

This was certainly the view of her hapless husband, a man who told me that he relied for extra income on "doin' a bit o' thievin'" of roofing lead from his employers. He tipped to one side as he walked, hindered by a slight limp, a legacy of childhood polio. He had also lost firm ground under his feet in the fen of his wife's malaise. He would have needed energy and imagination to deceive her. I thought her jealousy was delusional.

Thin and worried, propped against the pillows, a cotton nightdress fastened to the neck, she dismissed the fickle husband to the kitchen. Her teenage daughter took his place as chaperone. Jean was like her mother, anxious, appealing, not exactly pretty, slight, reliable. Mrs Sadler was discontented with the two older children, teenage boys, tall, awkward, scowling or grinning lads, too big for the house, who threw long shadows across the interiors of the small rooms as they clattered in the passages and doorways. She felt that they neglected her and used the house at their convenience. But Jean at fifteen, stamped with her mother's type of melancholy entreaty, and closely identified with her, tended her with sincere affection. Her adherence to her mother's side was born of her own fragility, but was not the less touching for that. Later, she raised her own family next door to her parent's home.

There was an allure about Mrs Sadler for a general practitioner susceptible to feminine helplessness. She placed herself under medical protection, and raised hopes for the gratification of therapeutic ambition. I responded to her needy submission. On this occasion, as on others, I thought I was unlikely to find much physically wrong. Many consultations at her home and at the surgery had convinced me that her problems were psychological and psychosomatic. The present diagnosis was established as period pains, dysmenorrhea. I prescribed more of her pain tablets.

Soon after I started in the practice, I took an interest in bodily complaints connected with underlying depression. Mrs Sadler and her older sister lived next door to one another, and often brought their children to the surgery together. Although her sister was under psychiatric supervision for depression, she was less receptive to psychological ideas. For this reason I found her less interesting than Mrs Sadler, who complained first about her bodily pains, and only when re-assured about them, talked of her unhappiness, and her obsessive, possessive jealousy.

She was eloquent in her own way, about her struggles. In the early days, I had referred her to a day clinic, where she was interviewed by a woman therapist. Touched by Mrs Sadler's naive readiness to give educated authority the benefit of her doubts, the doctor allocated her to a therapeutic group. She went twice, before she became convinced the others looked down on her. She may have been right, as probably the only person present plebeian in speech and dress. At that time psychotherapy was a middle class affair, and the only available clinic was in Hampstead.

Meanwhile, her sister made repeated attempts to do away with herself, in and out of mental hospital. Treated for profound and mystifying attacks of depression, by stupefying doses of drugs, and by electric shock therapy, she grinned mindlessly through it all, brisk and bright, hair blonded and cropped. Unlike her sister, she was unable to convey that of which she constantly spoke, her despair. There was certainly a close link with the loss of a two year old daughter in a cot death. She grinned in embarrassment when she got near to her pain about that, how they heard her "snoring" in her cot, and assumed the child was just sleeping late. Because the child sang in a clear sweet voice, on the potty, they called her 'Angel'. Now whenever she heard a child referred to as an angel . . . The mindless grin went, tears came.

When her son and daughter were teenagers, she finally escaped, by overdose, from whatever it was that tormented her.

I drove home from this visit to Mrs Sadler, through Drapers Lane, under the low railway bridge into Forest Road. The Council had completed their plan, later regretted, for a new estate on the site and in another five years the networks of intimate, but neglected dwellings would be cleared. Most residents were poor and old, some had lived there all their lives – their parents had rented the houses when they were built in the eighteen eighties. The most recent occupants were newly-arrived West Indian immigrants, with several families sharing the ancient plumbing. A few of the houses were owned, most let from private landlords,some had been destroyed by bombs in the war. Gaps were filled later with pre-fabricated bungalows, later replaced with incongruous pink villas, occupied by young couples.

Beyond the railway bridge lay a neater cleaner estate, with terraces in good repair, originally provided by the London North Eastern Railway Company for their employees at the local engine shed. From here the road gave access to the North Circular Road. Driving north past the reservoir, where the land shelves down to the lake, I passed an estate of red brick council houses, with gardens, and modern plumbing, built between the wars. Some of these were hit by German flying bombs in the nineteen forties and Mrs Sadler's mother and father were killed in one of those raids.

"I'll never forget it, doctor," she told me, in one of our talks, "There'd been a big air raid that night, we could tell from the shelter it wasn't far off. Next morning I was taking our Jim to my mother's as usual, she had him while I was at work. We were walking up from our house, and as soon as we crossed over at the lights, I could see there was trouble. Then I saw it was my Mam's house that had gone. Just a pile of rubble, and the police there. They said it was a direct hit, and asked me to identify my Dad. He was still alive, but he died later in hospital. They never asked me to identify Mam, they just showed me a ring with a red stone that she always wore, and an ear-ring. They never let me see her, because she wasn't all in one piece, she was blown so far. My two brothers were all right, one of them was just home on leave from the Navy."

She dabbed at her eyes with her handkerchief.

"I don't think my Jim has ever got over it, he was there with me, and only two years old. He said to me, 'Where's my Nan's front door gone, Mam?' It was after that I had my nervous breakdown."

Over four decades, I was to attend her many times with many minor, and some serious, complaints. She drank a lot of Guinness, and was agoraphobic. She rarely left the house by day without her daughter, or by night without her husband, long since cleared from the suspicion of infidelity . . .

I became deeply involved with that same Jim of hers, later, when he was thirty. We began to talk when he came to tell me, incoherently, about his left leg, which he claimed, ached so much that he was unable to go to work. He had developed huge varicose veins — like the trunk of a vine, twisted and knotted from ankle to groin. I did not at first connect this haggard dull man, several inches taller than myself, with the pallid, catarrhal, blank faced little lad brought to me so often by his mother in the fifties, or even with the skinny, distracted, restless twenty year old of the sixties who had fractured his left femur, and then re-fractured within a few days of discharge from hospital. This time he did not escape complications: thrombosis in the iliac and deep leg veins had forced the blood from his lower limb to return to the heart via these engorged superficial veins. To support them, he wore a heavy elastic stocking from ankle to groin, secured by a suspender belt round his waist.

20

Several medical and surgical opinions had been taken, but there was nothing more to be done. Pain in the leg exhausted him in anything but sedentary work, for which he had no aptitude, or qualification. Restless, dismayed, and sleepless, he had been on the telephone to the Samaritans. He wanted a certificate from me to claim National Insurance sickness benefit. I gave it to him, prescribed the sedatives he requested, and offered a weekly appointment to investigate what had happened to him.

I learned about his sleeplessness and how he wandered the streets at night; about his marriage seven years earlier to a widow whose husband had died in a car crash; there was jealousy at home between a stepdaughter and their own two daughters – he had to be careful in handling this, otherwise there would be a quarrel with his wife. He spoke of his childhood: his father's bad temper and his parents' quarrels with each other, of which I already knew something. He felt that he was now playing the same game with his children, being heavy handed and bad tempered. He had worked out in his own way this identification with a bad tempered father, and with this insight had come an effort to think about it and keep it under control. He spoke of his inability to hold down his job as a gatekeeper at a Council depot, how he thinks of taking an overdose like his mother, and of his aunt's suicide. He needed a drink before he could face anyone, couldn't even get to the doctors' without calling in at the pub first to steady his shakes.

One evening at home, the children had started to quarrel. He'd tried to restore peace, but failed, and there was a big row – him and his girls on one side, wife and stepdaughter on the other. He wasn't equipped for this, couldn't regain self control. When his wife's back was turned he'd taken a handful of his tranquilisers, downed his beer, and waited for oblivion. But one of the girls had seen him, and called her mother. He was taken to hospital, stomach washed out, and sent home the same night.

This long talk brought his wife down the next day to see me, dressed in widow's black, with Jim trailing behind. She looked middle-aged and thin, with a pinched, depressed look about her. She clipped her words short, through clenched uneven teeth, and was out of patience. I listened to her, while Jim sat depressed and guilty. I spoke a little about childhood passions

21

and said that it seemed the children's jealousy had led to the rupture between them. During the three-quarters of an hour of discussion, the ice melted, she expressed concern, and they went off together, friendly and agreeable. Jim found strength to return to his post.

In a few weeks he was back, leaden faced, garbed as always in jeans and donkey jacket. He couldn't keep up, had to report a savage dog to the authorities. He broke a sauce bottle at dinner table, when he couldn't stand the children arguing. He was expected to be at the back and the front of the premises at the same time. If any kids broke in, the boss would blame him. A couple of nights back, he had swallowed twelve sleeping tablets, after another row at home. His bad leg ached all the time.

Of the fractured femur, I knew only that three days after hospital discharge, he had broken it a second time. I had not before thought of a link with his father and his limp, perhaps because the listless glance and high cheek bones were so like his mother's. Now he struggled with his unruly mind to give me the story again.

On a freezing Christmas Day ten years ago, he had taken out his bicycle on the icy road.

"I remember ridin' down 'ill, fast as I could, thinkin' I didn't care what 'appened to me, and something did 'appen to me. I ran into a car door, just as this bloke was gettin' out."

He was in the orthopaedic ward for eight weeks, his fractured femur pinned, then out on crutches, to stay indoors. But he went out in the van with his uncle for a few drinks. (He waggled his right hand near his mouth by way of illustration, a reflex gesture with him, even if he spoke of his daughter having a drink of milk.) They were about to drive away from the pub, when Jim whistled at a girl. The fellow with her objected. Insults via the van window escalated into a tipsy challenge to a fight. Jim tried to leave the van to deal with the situation more effectively, fell over his crutches, and re-fractured the leg.

Did he think that "not caring what happened to me" could be suicidal? He shrugged, but looked at me with attention. He described his difficulty in staying at his job.

22

"I'm 'spected to write these reports, see, and me spellin's very bad, though I've taught meself to read since I lef' school"

I attended to my mental picture of Mrs Sadler twenty years younger, upset by Jim's school report. Behind her shuffled a twelve year old, flat faced and graceless. I recalled that I had wondered then about mental subnormality.

He pulled some scraps of paper from his jacket pocket:

"I carry some words round with me, case I need 'em for the reports. 'Ere's one, look . . ."

Each had its pencilled word: "locked" and "fence" and "catch".

"My Dad's a poor speller too, and 'e doesn't like me borrowing 'is dictionary, so I've bought meself a little 'un."

He pulled out of his other coat pocket a dog-eared Collins pocket dictionary.

Here was evidence of struggle to overcome both the handicap of his own dullness, and of a father possessive of the source of knowledge. I was interested in Jim's pre-occupation with the problem of delinquent intruders, and his responsibility to his superior for their control. He described with mounting indignation the leader of the gang who hung about the gate, a kid in a red pullover. But as a boy had he not been at that game himself? And, I thought to myself, his father also, in his younger days, filching lead from the Council?

He agreed, with a phantom grin.

"That's true. When I was a kid we'd jump on the trains down at the Junction, as they pulled out for Wycombe, and places. We'd walk around for a bit then when we got tired, we'd go to the police, and say we were 'ungry and didn't know 'ow to get 'ome. They'd give us some bread and butter, and send a message 'ome to Dad. 'E'd come and get us — and give us a wallopin'."

Our time was up. I gave him a sickness certificate with the diagnosis of depression, and invited him to come again the following week. He came eager to report that he had written

23

down that which he found so difficult to say. He handed me two sheets of soiled paper, torn from a cheap, lined writing pad. It looked like three stanzas of poetry, written in capital letters. The spelling was idiosyncratic, even with the help of his pocket dictionary:

> NOT ABLE
> TO STAND COMFORTABLE SHOURT TIME
> WITHOUT STRAIN AND SWELLING
> TO WALK A SHOURT DISTANCE WITH OUT A
>   SITE DOWN
> ACHING
> TO RUN OR RUSH ABOUT OR PLAY
>   FOOTBALL AND CRICKET
> TO RIDE A BIKE FOR A LONG TIME
>   ACHING
> TO CLIME STAIRS WITH OUT STRAIN
>   AND ACHING
> TO GO OUT WITH FAMILY FOR LONG
>   WALKS
> TO KEEP UP WITH FAMILY GOING
> ACHING SWELLING SHOPPING AND STANDING
> TO KNEE DOWN FOR SHOURT TIME
> TO CLIME LADDERS WITH OUT STRAIN
> ACHING   STRAIN
>
> NOT ABLE
> TO PUSH ANY THING HEAVY STRAIN
> TO WARK WITH OUT A SIT DOWN
> SWELLING ACHING. STRAIN
> TO GO OUT IN DAMP WEATHER
> AND FROST WITH OUT
> MY LEG FEELING VERRY
>   UNCOMFORTABLE
>
> TO SLEEP COMFORTABLE WITH LEG
> TO LAY ON ANY SIDE CANE ONLY LAY FLAT
> TO PLAY WITH CHILDREN WITH A BALL
>   OR RUNNING ABOUT

TO TAKE FAMILY TO CINEMA BECOURS
OF THE CRAMP SEATS
TO TAKE THE FAMILY TO THE CITY BECAUS
OF THE WALKING AND STANDING

NOT ABLE
TO SITE COMFORTABLE IN A SEAT FOR
 A LONG TIME ACHING
TO CARRY LOADS WITH OUT STRAIN
 AND SWELLING ACHING

TO KEEP UP WITH PEOPLE IN LIFE

This communication of suffering did not, I think refer solely to physical discomfort. In the following weeks I explored with him the concept of mental pain, its connection with depression and damaged objects, and the problems of reparation as a form of work that seemed to be beyond his capacities. This we did in a most elementary and basic form, but he was receptive to these complicated ideas and my efforts to show him the way I approached the problem of depression.

Sometimes his comments were startling in their directness, as when after remarking that his wife was jealous of him looking at women with large breasts, he told me that she wanted to change her doctor and register with the practice. He had warned her off by telling her "mine's full". I did offer to accept her on my list, and spoke of the problem he must have experienced as an infant in sharing his mother with others. We continued our weekly meetings at the end of the evening surgery for several months; then as he had returned to work, I decided to interrupt them.

But he came back after a while, again unable to work, and asked to continue the discussions.

He began with his inability to eat the food put in front of him because his mind was full of arguments with his supervisor, full of "cunts" and "fucks". Once when he was "on the dust" a mate called him a cunt. He lost his temper and threw a punch, but he frightened himself more than his antagonist, in case he lost control and did some damage he would regret.

"When I'm talkin' to the wife, I feel all right, then when I go to work, I get more and more talkin' to meself in this swearin'

25

way. It's funny, the other night I was at work and feelin'
terrible and I did think of ringin' you, but thought you would
think me stupid."

He spoke of a new job, assistant car park manager at the Town
Hall. He has to stop cars without a badge from parking. He feels
frightened of turning people away, stays in the hut, and avoids
the work.

"Part of me wants to get on with the job, part don't. I'm
supposed to ask the drivers in the car park which direction
they're goin'. If they give me a sharp answer I feel I want to
get back at 'em, then I get frightened at what I might do, so
I go back into the 'ut and let the boss get on with it."

After more weekly talks, he returned to the car park, on tablets
arranged in consultation with the hospital psychiatrist.

We continued to meet and talk at intervals for some years. He
came once in a panic, unscheduled. He roared in, out of
control, eyes wild, flat cheeks contorted. His lament burst from
him before he was properly through the door: he had a pain in
his belly and had been sick. He gave a hypochondriac's detailed
account of the agony of lying flat on his back, as he felt round his
stomach, and wondered if the pain would go up or down.

When I examined him, I could discover no obvious cause for
his pain. I knew his sister had given birth the day before. I
decided to risk putting to him the idea of an identification, a link
between his belly ache and his sister in labour.

The lament stopped and he looked at me with less amazement
than I expected, and remarked with composure that when his
wife had their baby he had the same symptoms.

"But it's not that, I don't think, doc. I think its 'cos I get so
cold at work in the car park, there's no 'eat in that little 'ut.
I don't even like to touch me own body, when it feels so cold.
Trouble is, I'm keen to do the right thing at work, but I can't
get any cooperation. I'm supposed to ask the drivers for their
pass, but they won't show 'em. My mate don't bother, but
then if anythin' goes wrong it's me what gets the blame.
There ain't enough to keep me busy either, and I don't like
'angin' around doing nothin'. I like to be busy."

"I seem to remember," I said cautiously, "that you always

used to feel that you got the blame at home when you and your brother were boys?''

"It's true. I always used to think Dad was my stepfather 'cos I always got blamed. I never did get on with young Stan. I never think about 'im now, don't even know where 'e is now, or when 'is birthday is.''

"Suppose your pain and the sickness goes back further than your wife's or sister's pregnancy, to when your mother was pregnant. You would be about four then. D'you think she might remember, and tell us, how you took the birth of Stan, when you were a boy?''

This conversation, reported to his mother, brought Mrs Sadler down the next evening.

"I'm worried about Jim, doctor. He says you think it's because he was jealous of Stan. I think it's more because of what happened when he was two, like I told you, about the air raid. He was really brought up by my mother, she used to have him when I was at work. He got a terrible shock that day I told you when we found her house hit by a rocket. And d'you know, he's never spoke about it from that day to this.''

Jim came back a few days later, as arranged. To my surprise he immediately told me two dreams from the night before.

"In the first dream I was a tiny naked baby with thick fluid pouring out of me mouth and behind, feeling very desperate. In the second one, I was still a baby, and glass got into me mouth, all splintered, and I was tryin' to claw it out.''

I encouraged him to think of associated ideas. He finally said,

"I'll tell you what it reminds me of, it's to do with Stan, and that feelin' that I always got the blame. There'd often be arguments at 'ome, when I was a kid I got frightened. I used to go next door to me Auntie's, the one who committed suicide, when there was trouble at 'ome. One night there was a row going on between Mum and Dad, and it woke me up. There was broken glass all over where my Mum 'ad smashed a bottle over Dad's back. I think you're right about the jealousy — it's like my kids at home, I always feel one of 'em gets the blame and 'as all the nerve troubles, while the other gets off free.''

27

On the other hand, he recalled he didn't like the teachers at school to speak to him kindly, he thought they were silly and wasting their time, he just moved his mouth saying yes, yes, yes, and waited for them to go away and talk to someone else. Was this me? He said he did think I was wasting my time when I spoke about his vomiting being due to his sister's pregnancy, although it was correct in connection with his wife's!

Jim changed his job to a road sweeper, and found it more suited to his restlessness.

Within a few weeks conflict with his conscience broke out again. Standing up all day made his leg ache, but it was his state of mind he found unbearable. He was tempted to "skive" like the others, they all seemed to finish early and get away with it; but on the day he tried it — he hid his dustcart and went to a cafe — he couldn't take the worry of being found out.

Sometimes he carried a bottle of cider in his barrow, to calm his worries, his obsessive over-conscientiousness.

"The foreman might say to me, 'Jim, just make sure the main road is clean, them side roads don't matter today. But then I 'ear in my 'ead people sayin' 'Roadsweeper, why aren't them side roads clean?'. Then I try to clean those too. I'm always like that in other jobs. I'd always try to carry more in the wheelbarrow than anyone else."

I spoke of the severity of a conscience that made life more of a misery for him than any foreman. He agreed and said that was when he started taking Largactil in big dosage to stop the panic. He agreed that when he stopped work, and had nothing to occupy his mind, but just brooded on all his problems, his depression deepened; after some persuasion he agreed to return to work instead of taking the sick certificate he had come for.

I heard nothing more until some months later he staggered into the consulting room, leaving the door open for his agitated wife to close.

"Sorry, doc. I've 'ad a drink. I 'ad to do it. I was gettin' too excited again. Can't speak anymore just now."

He sat down, head in hands, while his wife talked: there had been a row at work; the foreman had wanted to change Jim's

28

barrow for one that didn't wheel properly; Jim refused it, lost control, and bashed in his barrow with his shovel, so that no-one else could use it, stormed out, crashed into a lamp-post, broke his spectacles and cut his eyebrow.

"I can talk now doc. My trouble is I can't stand up to people bullyin' me. I just shut up and walk away. I wasn't goin' to let them do it to me today, but if I do stand up to people then I feel guilty. I can't bear the idea that I've hurt anyone, I'd rather hurt meself. That's my trouble. I love work, but I can't bear responsibility. I tell you, I worked for fourteen years in the sewers. I stood in those trenches killin' meself, but he was such a good foreman, I enjoyed it so long as I didn't 'ave the responsibility. The trouble is there's no foreman around like that anymore."

Jim, the author of those stanzas on pain, was always able to arouse my sympathy. Amongst other things I think I said that he bashed himself in, just as he bashed the barrow in. They left after a few more minutes, calmer. I had the thought that I was in some way connected with that foreman . . . .

He told me once that he was a "spare man" at work. As his work record was so bad, he either replaced men off sick, or was sent along to help somebody else.

His foreman wanted him to work in another part of the borough, further from his home. He protested that he felt frightened being in a strange area, and he was too far from home to call in for a smoke or a cup of tea. He declared that he was no longer able to eat in a cafe, where he was overcome by panic. His wife came to see me. She wanted something done, life at home was impossible, she couldn't stand it: he made her take charge of his money, so that he wouldn't spend it all in the pub, then when she refused to give him what he wanted, he would be furious and swear at her and the children. The hospital psychiatrist, who had earlier discharged him, as Jim drank with the sedatives "to stop his mind from racing," agreed to see him again and he was admitted for some weeks, but there was no change in the situation when he came home.

There followed a period of time when I lost contact with Jim, as the psychiatrist at the hospital took over responsibility for him. He was now on very heavy dosage of sedatives and sleeping tablets, which he supplemented by alcohol. He hung on at work, between admissions to the psychiatric ward for over-dosing complicated by quarts of Guinness, usually a sequel to rows at home.

When he came to me again, he asked for my help in returning to the car park job, which now seemed preferable to street cleaning. His list of problems included those arising from his leg, his fear of being knocked down by traffic, his weak bladder — worries about finding a toilet — his anxiety about leaving his barrow unattended when he went to the cafe. His council employers were reluctant. He had come to the end of his working life at forty two.

Then he discovered that the responsibility for the collection of a sickness benefit certificate could be delegated to his diligent sister, Jean, until I suggested that he come himself each month so that our contact could be maintained.

He hoped he had reached a pain-free haven, free from conflict, responsibility, and the terror of doing some harm. But there was a final act to be played out. I heard from him first of his wife's mounting intolerance to his befuddled, depressed way of life, then that he had been admitted to hospital with an overdose: she had announced her intention to leave him.

After the divorce, his plan to have the custody of his ten year old daughter fell through. One day he persuaded her to come home to her grandparent's with him. When she ran back to her mother, he downed several large rums and then slashed his wrists. He was re-admitted to hospital.

There was indignation when his ex-wife was sighted with another man, more when she re-married. Then, honour satisfied, Jim and his parents settled down together. From the flat next door, where she lived with her husband and children, Jean, continued to care for them all, and to carry the responsibility the others found so hard to bear . . . .

When Mrs Gloria Wall was a teenager, she left school and learned to assemble wireless sets. She was a girl who mixed bashfulness and flirtation in apt proportions for the provocation of teasing, which caused her to blush prettily. When she was twenty she met Fred at a dance. He was Irish, but had come to London as a boy. He was the only son of an ex-regular Army sergeant, and like his four sisters had been born in India. Gloria and Fred Wall were married in 1939, just before the war.

Then he became ill with renal tuberculosis and was in hospital on and off throughout the war. No children were conceived, he was sterile. They quarrelled a lot, and she remembered her mother's warning "God help you if you marry that Fred!" After each quarrel she would run back to the little house where she was born, to be consoled by her mother. This was about half a mile away, in a terrace which faced a cemetery, though the graves were shielded from view by a high brick wall. Gloria was the seventh child in a family of ten, and she felt that no-one took much notice of her as a child, partly because she was not as pretty as her older sisters. Her father liked a drink, and quarrelled with her mother. When he died, he was buried at the cemetery opposite. Her mother socialized amongst convivial friends once her husband and ten children were off her hands.

Mrs Wall's first depressive breakdown came after fifteen years of marriage. She complained to the psychiatrist that her husband didn't acknowledge her sacrifices for him, that he was an extravagant gambler, that he was unfaithful, although he denied it and accused her of being a flirt. In a mental hospital for three months, she submitted to electric shock therapy, until her husband became ill again with tuberculosis and sent for her. He now added to his accusations that she was mad, a hospital case. He developed tubercular abscesses under the skin, and was admitted to hospital, where she visited him every day.

He recovered and they continued their life together. During these uneasy years of truce, they registered at the practice. Mrs

Wall was tall, slim, elegant and looked young for forty eight. Dark haired, with a fringe of ringlets on a handsome forehead, her amber eyes glittered, her glance was first combative, and then pleading, assisted by an expressive lipsticked, petulant mouth. She wore pendant earrings and a small cross hung from a gold neckchain. Discreetly coloured nails drew attention to graceful fingers. She talked well, and had numerous complaints: backache, indigestion, gynaecological anxieties. Her manner was engaging, by turns flirtatious, appealing, self critical, aggressive:

> "I'm horrible, doctor," she would say, "I'm proud, that's why I don't like asking for help, why I don't ask my husband to take me out. Perhaps it's my mother — she was good to us, don't misunderstand me — but there were so many of us it was no use asking for anything, no-one took any notice. I feel mothers should give up everything for their children, I'm sure I would if I had children. My mother had a baby every two years for twenty years, and she was going to have a good time as soon as she could. We were left at home then, she was always going out to a dance!"

Mr Wall was sick at home, moping, and ruminating, confused by a mixture of pain from his renal tuberculosis, and from hypochondria, difficult to separate into its component parts. When I visited him, with Gloria's version of his character in mind: "obstinate and selfish," he was in bed, smoking a cigarette, as he watched the racing on the television, with the Daily Mirror at hand.

He looked unhealthy, but not ill. Lanks of grey hair were controlled with hair-cream, except for a few untidy strands stuck out at the nape. The complexion of his triangular shaped face was rough with old acne scars, and his chin was deeply cleft. When he smiled, his furrowed brow and deep set eyes of grey steel, took no part, only his lips.

He was suspicious of me, one of his wife's men, and I found him pre-occupied with his own pain. I cautiously sounded out the possibility that some of it might be connected with depression, but he would have none of that, and my heart wasn't in it. The hospital had just discharged him, able to return to work, but he disagreed and wanted me to certify him unfit. It was my responsibility to enquire into the impasse, but he refused to talk about anything other than his tuberculosis — and his wife's shortcomings.

Finally he agreed to another opinion, provided it took place at home — he insisted he was too ill to travel. I called in a sympathetic physician, relieved to share the responsibility, and it was useful for the specialist to see him in his home setting. His opinion was that the hospital discharge report from his colleague was correct. He thought the refusal to leave the house, apart from short evening visits to the pub and the betting shop, were not malingering, one could hardly say that of a man who had so much illness, he agreed that the man was a difficult character, and regretted he could not be more helpful. The impasse was only resolved when Fred Wall took early retirement from his job, and was free to spend his time as he wished, while Gloria continued at work in a small electronics factory.

Then, Fred won five hundred pounds on the football pools, and refused Gloria a share. After a row, she took an overdose at four in the morning. While she was in hospital, her husband came to see me, personable in a smart brown raincoat and sporty cloth cap, which he politely removed, before sitting down. He anticipated that I would blame him for his wife's behaviour, and was guarded with me. He sat by the side of the desk, smiled knowingly and stroked his chin:

"I know you take her side, doctor, but you don't know her like I do. After I won that money she gave me no peace, she thought I ought to spend it all on her. She's very jealous, she doesn't like me to have anything to do with my sisters. I've bought them a few things, clothes and perfume, not as much as I spent on her. Don't mistake me, I love my wife, but she's got this idea into her head about me and another woman, when it's really the other way round. You know her, you see her, she's an attractive girl, and dresses well. All her family are the same, two of her sisters have gone off with other men."

"She told me you wanted to have an evening out every week without her ....?"

"Of course. I like going to the pub for a drink, she doesn't. I've got a lot of friends and she says she doesn't like them.

33

She'll tell you that she doesn't want me to bet, but has she said that if I'm too ill to go round to the betting shop she goes for me? Gloria's a good talker, she's a clever girl, and I know the way she gets round you doctors, and puts me in the wrong. And I'll tell you this, I don't think it's right the way she's given all those tablets. She can't get to sleep now without a couple of pills. I've got myself to think about, what good does it do me, if I'm always worried about how many she's taken? Can't you do something for her, besides pills?"

"She told me that you haven't spoken to each other for six weeks . . . .?"

"That's her doing. She began by sulking 'cos I wouldn't give her half the money I won. I told her it was my winnings and she could have something she wanted, but there was no law to say I had to give her half. She went back to her mother's place again, I've had that all our married life. I can't stand this sort of thing anymore, I'm not a fit man, I have to go to the hospital every six weeks with my kidneys. My back plays me up since I tried to go back to work on your advice. You think I exaggerate and it's all in the mind. That's not what they tell me in the hospital. As a matter of fact I told the specialist that my G.P. thinks it's all in my head, and he said that was ridiculous. There's a T.B. abscess in the pelvis you can see on the X-rays."

"What I said was that there was the possibility that some of your pain . . . ."

"Well, I'll tell you they don't agree with you at the hospital and I don't either. It's Gloria that's mixed up, not me. That's what I tell you and what I've told the solicitor. I'm going to do what I should have done years ago, I'm going for a divorce. When I told her, she said she was sorry, and could we try again, but I told her that I couldn't stand this sort of life any more, and I wouldn't change my mind. That's why she took those damned pills. I don't think you should give her any more, I don't think it's right. She needs proper treatment."

Mrs Wall was discharged from hospital a few days later, but they both wanted something more to be done. I arranged a consultation at a psychotherapy clinic which sometimes admitted patients, and the consultant agreed to take her.

I called to see her after a week, and as she was at lunch, I spoke to the resident doctor. He was a serious young man, in an unbuttoned white coat, about thirty, slight, with small soft hands quickly withdrawn from our handshake. His curly black hair was thin on the crown, and through the limpid lenses of gold framed spectacles, the magnified irises of his pale blue eyes flickered. He addressed me academically:

"Clinically she presents as an immature personality, possibly with hysterical features, and there are also obsessional and paranoid traits. My consultant thought she would require ECT but I have given him my reasons for postponing it. I don't myself advocate shock therapy, it's the older psychiatrists who still use it. Considering the information he got from her on the day of admission, I think his decision was right, but I have been more fortunate in getting her confidence, which enabled me to discover some psycho-pathologically valid material from her childhood. She is attending my therapeutic group three times a week and participating well in the occupational therapy .... ah, her she is. Gloria, your doctor has come to see you. You're lucky to have a G.P. who visits you, we see them here all too seldom."

"Oh, doctor," groaned Mrs Wall when he was out of sight, "How long do I have to stay here? It's terrible! Well, I shouldn't say that, everyone is so kind, I'm not complaining about that. You know me, doctor, I'm grateful for people trying to help me, but this place is making me worse. The other patients upset me, when I look at them I don't feel I'm that ill, I want to help them, poor devils. I'm not mad, am I? I want to be in my little home with my poodle. Fred's been to visit me every day and he needs me. Can't you ask them to let me go home?"

"The psychiatrist says he thinks you ought to stay at least six weeks."

"I couldn't stay that long! You've seen my flat, how clean everything is. You know me, I love to have everything feminine and dainty, lace, flowers. At least I did 'til I got this depression. Now I can't be bothered. I can't eat the food here and I can't sleep without the drugs. What am I going to do? Fred wants me home. He misses me now I'm not there to look

35

after him. It's always been like that, he needs me and I suppose I need him."

She laid her hand on my arm and wept a little.

We were in the sitting room of a mental institution. All was alien to intimacy: the lethargic atmosphere, institutional green moquette furnishings, newspaper agent magazines, grey linoleum, hospital blue paint, chairs arranged in line. The unconscious patronage of many of the staff added to her own sense of helplessness, the company of the confused and dejected leached away what was left of hope. All these were an obstacle to recovery, I thought, when she would be better served by a struggle at home with her problems. Although she complained of loss of interest in her flat, and in her appearance, I never saw either neglected.

I agreed to ask for her discharge from the hospital, but proposed we should meet once a week, to contain and explore the problem. Her husband now accepted this mode of therapy with good grace, but not before she had brought him to me to represent all her own possible objections, and suspicions of my competence. After this he was much less provocative and peevish, and expressed some gratitude for the trouble I had taken with them since they had registered with me.

Thus started two years of weekly talks, from which it became clear that there was a childlike part of her personality that was very negative. This was a part of her self that it was convenient to split off into her husband, who voiced for her all her misgivings about my interest in them.

"No, it not like that!" was a meaningless, automatic response to every suggestion I made, as she continued to value my time and attention. We went over the details of her childhood and her relationships to her nine brothers and sisters, and the realisation came to her that she had lost, or mislaid, her feeling of affection for her mother and father. Her little girl flirtatiousness was also unmistakable. There was one occasion when she developed a painful thrombosis of a little vein, near her anus, an external haemorrhoid. When I insisted on the presence of the nurse during my examination, she protested,

"But doctor, you know I trust you!"

When she understood that on the contrary, it was I who did not trust her not to giggle with exaggerated embarrassment, she was offended at first, but quickly decided not to make an issue over it. This was, I think, significant. She thereafter struggled to some extent to overcome the artificiality of her girlish coyness with me, always an obstacle to serious discussion.

We settled into a routine at the end of the Friday evening surgery, an unpredictable point in time. But she never failed her appointment, and endured without complaint the awkwardness of the waiting room, where she sat until everyone had been attended to. This was not so easy for someone of her pride, but she was helped by the tact and friendliness of the receptionist.

As we talked, and attempted to contain and comprehend her disquieted feelings, she sought to escape from the meaning of her thoughts and actions by protean changeableness. Now languorous and mocking with an elegant arm draped over the chair, then perched aggressively on the edge of the seat, distrustful of my sincerity, the next moment on her feet, histrionically offended, or if she felt there was no way out, slumped into dejection and self-denigration. She was never late, rarely overtly grateful but clearly very dependent.

After twelve months of this, Fred Wall came in with chest pain. He was friendly, cheerful, almost joyous. When I diagnosed a coronary thrombosis his smile did not go away. I wondered, as he grinned slyly throughout the consultation, if he thought his suffering might be at an end. In his thirty year struggle against tuberculosis he had lost a kidney and testicles, besides many painful other complications. Despite my warnings, he would agree to nothing but rest at home, and died two weeks later in the street outside his home. I was shocked, not only by his death and the anxiety that I might have done more to prevent it, but also by an unmistakable sense of relief, so tangible, that I did not know how I could face Mrs Wall.

She was baffled at first, as if Fred had bested her even in this. Then, stunned by remorse, she gazed for hours out of her sitting room window onto the street where he died, and envied the dead, who were happy. She had the poodle put down, their baby. Was it just spite, or had she decided to join her husband and continue the battle on the other side?

She began to bring dreams to our sessions: *her husband fell out*

37

of his coffin and the house was a terrible mess. A policeman appeared and said "There is nothing anyone can do". Another was a nightmare from which she woke screaming. She phoned at 2 a.m. and sobbed that she dreamed that Fred had tried to pull her into the grave.

With recovery, she found a muted note of melancholy that was bearable, but her familiar mockery and defiance mingled with sadness and remorse.

"If you cure me now I won't be able to stand it, you'll be all pompous and think how clever you've been. But you're lucky, you don't know what it's like. You've got a wife and children. Look at me, I'm fifty five now, look at the changes. Fred waited until it was too late for me to think of marrying again to have children. I don't blame him, I don't blame myself, but you can't know how I feel now. I feel really mean, you'd be shocked. I'm sure I'd hurt anyone if I thought I could get better."

She gave me a nasty look. I said that I expected that she had in mind other women's husbands, including me, and that the thought must have been there when as a little girl, and "on the shelf" she contemplated her mother and father. We had often discussed her feelings of painful singleness and hurt pride as a child, but now she rose from the chair and with hauteur, mixed with self mockery, pronounced,

"If you're going to say things like that, I shan't come again!"

She did continue to come, of course, and in fact that meaningful exchange remained in both our minds, and helped the process along. She decided to return to work, but not to her old job. She chose unskilled, badly paid unpleasant labour in a grubby factory, and then grumbled at being degraded by the dirt, and the coarseness of the factory hands. Unpredictable in everything but instability, in one session she would recall her misery as a child, boast of tomboy provocations, weep for her husband, and confess that she had received flowers from a married man.

This last item emerged from hiding, in an account of her husband's illness during the war years. She had encouraged this man many years ago, she said, because he was able to obtain food off the ration which Fred desperately needed. Now, all these years later, he had hired a detective to find her, discovered she was a widow, and wouldn't take 'no' for an answer. She showed me the card that came with the flowers as proof that she was telling the truth, said she had become too dependent on me, and that it was time to stop.

She also wanted referral to hospital, on the grounds that I said everything was "nerves". This return of her negativism came at a time when I had been called in by one of her sisters to attend their mother, who had sprained her ankle. The old lady lived alone in the terrace house, opposite the grave-yard, but the sister was a close neighbour, and carried most of the day to day responsibility for her. She had slowly deteriorated in her mobility in the last year, and Mrs Wall had found her thoughts more occupied with her. She remembered past kindness, more than old resentments. She talked of how two of her brothers and one of her sisters had fallen out with the mother, and no longer visited her.

We both recognised and spoke of the connections this emotional turbulence made with our own complicated relationship.

"Fred lies with his mother now," she said one night, "I have no-one but you."

She wept quietly and appealed to me not to abandon her. Before I went away for a summer holdiay, she left a small gift, too bashful to hand it to me in person. When we resumed in the autumn, she spoke of her love of her father, then moaned about how unreliable I was in my judgement of her chest pains, and perhaps of Fred's heart attack. She sought a comfortable state of mind, while assailed with a spectrum of pains: hopelessness, hypochondria, unhappiness, suspicion, gratitude, jealousy, remorse. Finally a wistful melancholy enabled her to bear the thought of her ill luck in marriage, and of the babies she might have borne, and she admitted that her infidelity came first, her husband's came later, in revenge.

She was frightened, and angry with me as the agent of her pain. She likened me to Dr. Fu Manchu, a film character of whom she was terrified as a child. But self respect returned on the tide of her remorse, she gave up the hated factory job, and trained as a receptionist, a post which suited her personality and in which she found satisfaction and popularity.

The first anniversary of Fred's death came, and after this, thoughts about how long we were to continue. The sessions helped her to bear regret, and revived vitality, and though she feared relapse, was not insensitive to the needs of others. Each Friday evening, she saw the reality of the much crowded waiting room. She felt lucky to receive so much attention, but uncomfortable and guilty, and this time her genuine bashfulness, when she asked to continue beyond the second anniversary of her husband's death, was touching. We agreed that after this, the routine appointments should stop.

Childish sexual confusion and excitement now contained, she felt secure enough to speak openly of her gratitude and affectionate dependence on the work we had done together. This time her infant needs had been met with some of those satisfactions of which she had felt deprived as the seventh of ten children. Her responsiveness increased my own feelings of affection for her. Regret for the wasted years, was offset by the freedom to please herself now Fred was gone. She was not free from worries about her health and nagging hypochondria, and when another married man appeared briefly on the scene, her periods stopped. The idea of raising a child was unthinkable, would I help her to a termination? But she was fifty six. It was the menopause.

Her mother, in the family home opposite the cemetery, lived contentedly amongst a diminished band of contemporaries. A drink in the pub, bingo, and family gossip were her pleasures. Other needs were supplied by ten children anxious to be dutiful, each in their own way. When she broke a hip and her mind wandered into the confusion of dementia, a place was found for her in an old people's home. Mrs Wall visited and comforted her, and when after two years her mother died, she commented that her mother had enjoyed a good life and a long life, and in many ways had been more fortunate that herself. She had experienced guilt and remorse after Fred's death, but now she was rational and calm. This grown up reasonableness was disturbed by turbulence from a more childlike level: her heart rate slowed to 48 and the drop in blood pressure made her faint.

We now met only occasionally, whenever she felt the need. When she came, it was with physical symptoms that she presented herself. I understood that she did not like to presume that my interest in her would continue as before. But I enjoyed her visits and her dramatic gift for parodying the foibles of the men in her office — and her own. The "boy friend" had given up the pursuit, but she delighted in her popularity with the men at work, whom she pretended were quite unable to resist her charms. Yet, I noticed that at each anniversary of Fred's death she came with a complaint of abdominal pain. When I commented on this, she was offended:

"It worries me that you always say it's my nerves, I think to myself that you may be making a mistake, and then I'll die. Whatever I say you always twist my words, though you'll say its me that twists yours. I think of the way poor Fred died in the street, I'd hate that, to go like that unnoticed. It was different with my mother. She had a full life with us ten children. Then she enjoyed herself, and we looked after her right to the end — at least some of us did. Some of my brothers and sisters were awful, and hardly saw her at all at the end."

She wanted to express hostility, be reassured that nothing would change between us, then she could feel better again.

I was always careful to investigate her physical complaints, acutely aware, in fact, of the pitfall of calling everything "nerves". She had been investigated several times at the hospital, and it was some years before the abdominal pain was finally put down to gallstones and she submitted reluctantly to surgery.

"Really I'm fine again now," she commented that Christmas. "it was cancer I was frightened of, like my sister Joan. But I've had a wonderful Christmas. I'm ever so popular at work. I got more presents than anyone else!"

She smiled at her own childlike pleasure and preened herself, drawing attention to her tall slender figure and shapely legs.

"I go to keep fit classes. All the other women there are fat or recovering from pregnancy. I'm probably one of the oldest there, but I can do a high kick and I look smashing in a leotard. Well, you know me doctor, I'm a bitch! I have to be in charge of everybody. At the office party the boss offered to

41

take me home. I called out to everyone 'This is how I do things, I get the boss to take me home!' "

As usual, her self mockery covered her pain about other women's pregnancies. She consoled herself with her eternal youthfulness, although she was now sixty-two.

"I've always been like this, doctor" She was keen always to anticipate what she thought I was about to say. "I've always been active. When I was a little girl I used to dash out of the house and do handstands and cartwheels. If I was missing, the neighbours would say to my Mum, 'If you're looking for Gloria she's upside down, standing on her hands, with her feet against the cemetery wall!' "

The sombre note sounded again: in the cemetery opposite her childhood home, were father, husband and mother.

"There is something I want to tell you. The other day coming home from work, I saw a funny little woman in the street, just near my place. She looked so peculiar, such funny shabby clothes, not a friend in the world, a real lost soul. I couldn't just walk past her as I would have done once. I stopped and talked to her. I thought of you and what you'd say, I don't know what, something about my once being like that myself."
"Or perhaps of your mother when she was ill?"
"Anyway, I asked her if she'd like to come round for tea one Sunday, and she came, and watched the telly. She's what I call a Mary Ann: a single woman who never tells you her age. She told me she was going to an office party, everything she had on was so tatty, I gave her an old coat. Well, I say an old coat, but you know me I look after things, it was a jolly nice coat." She giggled. "You know, the funny thing was she told me in confidence how old she was. She thought she was older than me, and she was only fifty-six! Anyway, she said she'd have to pay me for the coat and she left an envelope for me a few days later with ten pounds in it. I was surprised, she went up in my estimation. She's so funny, she told me later that if I hadn't given her a coat she was going to wear her mother's, and she's been dead for fifteen years!'

It was three months before I saw her again. She made herself at home in the consulting room, taking time to disrobe of an elegant coat, and space for a mannered removal of a silk headscarf, before she subsided languidly into the chair by the desk, with a rustle of skirt and a show of leg. I wondered what unconscious force was bringing her to me this time. She complained unconvincingly of catarrh, but when I asked her for news of "Mary Ann", she came to life:

"She comes for tea every few weeks now, I was surprised, one day it was really cold and wet but there she was on the doorstep. Mind you, she's not so daft, she expects little things from me now, skirts and so on, and she doesn't offer to pay. I worry about her, I'm sure she doesn't get enough to eat. She doesn't spend enough on clothes even to keep herself warm in this weather, though she is working and earns a decent wage. She's funny you know, I catch her out in little fibs. She said her father died when he was ninety, and then the other day, she said eighty!" She giggled at what was coming next. "You can't tell lies to a liar!" She threw back her head and laughed with delight. "I gave her some meat pie to eat although she says she's a vegetarian and she wasn't all that keen. She said she can't eat anything that comes from having been killed. I said to her, 'Well, you just ate a poached egg!' I'm wicked to tease her. The next time she came she asked for cauliflower cheese!"

She sobered up suddenly, and looked downcast.

"Oh, doctor, my mother! When I think how she used to walk round to our house when Fred was in hospital! She'd say 'I've just come with some cigarettes for Fred, tell him they're from me.' And I was short with her, 'cos I knew she'd want me to walk her back home. I do feel terrible about that, but I suppose I was always in a hurry to catch the bus for visiting time. Poor Fred, he didn't have much of a life did he doctor? It seems funny now, life seems to go so quickly. We met at a dance, you know. I was always keen on keep fit and acrobatic dancing and that's how we met, at a dance . . . . ."

4   Boxed in

The old surgery stood where three roads met. A small traffic island was a vortex around which swirled traffic, men, women and children. Workers, pensioners, idlers, shoppers, pram pushers, and youngsters of all sizes, hurried, limped and skipped across the junction, as they dodged the millrace of cars, buses, vans and lorries, surging from three directions.

The turbulence of dust, fumes, and the debris of the street, left a precipitate in the surgery garden. Old newspapers, cigarette ends, beer cans and paper bags mingled with the fallen leaves of the lime trees planted nearly a century ago when the house was built, at the end of a spacious terrace, modified to meet the requirements of the first medical man to put up his plate in that area.

On fine evenings, drinkers spilled out of the Chained Bull, on the opposite side of the High Road, and some crossed over, pints in hand, to perch on the surgery garden wall: their farewells at closing time ("G'night Bill, G'night Tom, G'night Bill") then irritated would-be sleepers trying to drop off in the bedroom just above their heads. The old Victorian pub was a gloomy mammoth, convex and fleshy on a wide arc of the curve of the road. Seen from the surgery the cavernous bars intimidated, rather than invited.

Rarely, the publican sent across for medical help: someone stabbed, or dead from a heart attack. Most of the calls were to attend depressed and homesick young domestics or barmaids, come to London from rural Ireland and accommodated in dusty, high ceilinged, narrow bedrooms in the furthest recesses of the pile. I would be led past Cerberus, a discontented Alsation guarding a back entrance, through a gloomy labyrinth, up and down stairs and along corridors, until in a shadowy room, a collapsed adolescent, neglected and scared, lay in soiled sheets wondering how she had ended up so far from home.

From the other direction, traffic flowed downhill past the parish church. There was a sharp left hand curve which concealed the junction ahead. As drivers braked, they found the approach obstructed by parked cars on all sides. An impatient queue of vehicles might bring them to a halt before the petrol pumps of Wood's Garage, opposite the surgery on the other corner site. Cars moving in and out of the forecourt and to and from the lock-ups and workshops behind, met any random glance through the net curtains of the consulting room window.

Post-war waves of immigration from the West Indies were beginning. Re-development of the area was on the drawing board. Shops had begun to change hands, the Odeon had started Bingo sessions, many residents planned to move out. A meeting was called by the local Health Authority, at which family doctors were invited to surrender their individual surgeries, and combine in a health centre to be constructed at the top of the only steep road in the neighbourhood. No-one was interested. It was pointed out how difficult that site would be for the disabled and women with prams. The project was shelved. Business at garage, pub and surgery continued as before.

Two middle aged brothers Cyril and Jim Wood, owned the garage. Four petrol pumps, with a little kiosk between for the attendant, were kept busy. Behind the forecourt, the founder of the business, the father of the present proprietors, had designed and contructed a plain flat-faced two story brick structure, with office space, and a house for his family. This was still the home of his widow and her elderly companion, a bashful lady who had answered the advertisement for a ladies companion and house-keeper. She played a self-effacing but indispensable role in the family organisation.

I had an account there myself. The Wood brothers seemed cool with me at first, when I first introduced myself as the new assistant, from the practice across the road. Then, from several sources, I discovered that my predecessor in the post had been less than prompt in paying his bills, and preferred to spend his money at the pub, and that the turnover in assistants to my future partner had recently been brisk. Our relationship improved after I survived my first year there.

The Woods were not patients of the practice. The sons with their wives and children lived elsewhere, but for their mother, home was the garage at the road junction. Experienced and benevolent, pleasant and well provided for, from her sitting room she presided equitably over her sons' partnership. Some days, as I filled up with petrol at the pumps, she waved as she alighted from a Rover, a Jaguar, or a Daimler, made available to her as it passed through the hands of the firm. Her deferential driver, a retainer from the old days, when not required by his mistress, helped out at the kiosk, washed cars, and did odd jobs for the brothers. We got on nodding terms, as she was getting in or out of a limousine, and I was filling up at the pumps.

One day she had an attack of palpitation, and sent across the road for me. I found she had an irregular heart beat, which settled with a small dose of digitalis. After this she sometimes came over to consult me. She said her own doctor, whom she attended privately, was commited to hospital work, rather than general practice. She was fond of him, had attended him for the last twenty five years, but like her he was no longer young, and was reluctant to visit. She hesitated to disturb him at night. Would I be willing to attend her, if she became ill at home, without the other having to know, as she didn't want him offended? I agreed to this collusive arrangement and thereafter she consulted me occasionally either at the surgery, or in her home behind the forecourt.

Cyril Wood, the elder brother, balding, bespectacled, reticent to the point of unsociability, presided over reception and the book-keeping, in dark suit and waistcoat. The prevailing mood there was slow and obsessive. Jim Wood with hair awry, hands and overalls coated with oil, was the skilled mechanic, to be found with his head under a bonnet, in the workshop. There, in the sheds at the back, he kept company with the tenants of other sheds, body shops, paintshops. The firm's activities there were bustling, busy, helpful, and cheerful.

The brothers each had a son, a third generation to carry on the family business.

Soon after my last conversation with her, the old lady sent for me again, but it was her elderly and fragile companion whom I found unconscious, and who died next day.

When I heard from her, again it was about one of her grandsons. Roy was twenty, and I saw him most days of the week across the road, out of my window, or when I filled up, or my car was serviced. He was the son of the older brother, the one in reception. I first met him when he was only eighteen

47

months old. His parents lived nearby in those days, and their own doctor not being available (the same one!) they called me late at night, because they couldn't stop Roy from screaming. I was new to the practice then and somewhat raw, and had never seen a night terror like it.

I was confronted with a muscular infant, their first, who had grappled himself to the rail of his cot, and who would not under any circumstances be persuaded to lie down. I hadn't met the mother before, she was rarely at the garage, and she was content to leave it to her husband to explain. Both parents were white with anxiety, while little Roy glared like a demon, and yelled in terror at any attempt to get near him: he was not to be approached or comforted in any way. I realised that my options were very limited, that his nearly demolished parents distrusted my competence, and that I was unlikely to calm any of them much. I took my time in the examination of the child as best I could, tried to re-assure all three that there was no serious physical cause for his behaviour, left a sedative for what I said was probably a nightmare, and came home shaken by the experience.

Roy grew up, a round faced, sturdy little fellow, precocious in self-confidence and condescension. He was often to be seen around the garage where he made a second home with his grandmother. At five, he played around the pumps, at ten he would try his hand in the repair shop. At fifteen he was a plump adolescent who planned to leave school: he wasn't much of a success there and would in any case be apprenticed to the trade. His cousin, the son of the other brother, and the same age as Roy, was a good looking, quiet youth, whose education went ahead without difficulty and who was also to be seen in the workshop, and around the garage, industriously learning his trade. There was a friendly rivalry, between the boys who were expected to succeed their fathers in the business.

But now, his grandmother told me, Roy was ill, had been for months and they were all very worried about him, had I not heard? His father, in reception, whom I saw frequently about the garage, restricted his communication with me to the business of sending me a monthly account. His inert features rarely expressed emotion, and the medical connection had not been renewed in the twenty years since he had called me to the house. He and his family had long moved to an outer suburb and saw a family doctor there.

The old lady was not satisfied. About twelve months ago, she said, Roy was on his way back from Cambridge one evening, in his car. He was engaged to a young lady there, and had made the journey many times. But on this occasion he found himself unable to complete the journey home, and pulled up in a lay-by, too frightened to go any further. There he stayed for about an hour, before returning to Cambridge. From his fiancée's home, he phoned for his father to come and fetch him.

According to his grandmother's story, his parents took him the next day to the doctor, who said it was depression and anxiety and sent him to a psychiatrist. He insisted that Roy break off the engagement. This seemed strange to me, but I realised that I was hearing of the events between Roy and the psychiatrist at least at third hand; Roy apparently put up no resistance to this idea. There followed a series of consultations and discussions, with Roy failing to respond to prescribed tablets and electric shock therapy. Months had gone by, and Roy still would not drive himself anywhere, in case it happened again. It all seemed quite absurd in a boy whose whole life was cars and driving.

His grandmother wanted to know what I thought of this story. If she could get him to agree to it, would I talk to him? She had not consulted his parents, had decided to speak to me first. Roy made no move to contact me, until several weeks later, when he came up to me as I filled up with petrol.

When he came to see me he described the same incident related by his grandmother. He had been returning to London, eighteen months ago from a visit to his fiancée of four weeks, when he began to feel panicky and pulled up in a lay-by.

"Then I felt I couldn't move from there. I can't explain it. It was horrible. Just as if I was shut up in a little box."

He rested and then found that he was able to go back to his fiancée's home, from where his father collected him.

Since then he had been unable to drive his car anywhere except to and from work. For any other journey he needed an escort, before he would take the wheel. This was baffling because cars were his obsession, his only interest. He had

49

become more and more depressed, wept unaccountably, had broken off his engagement, and was now heavily dependent on tablets. He wanted to stop them but was frightened that without them he would have a similar breakdown. He had been terrified by the electric shock therapy and after two treatments had refused any more.

He maintained that he had never been depressed before, although he remembered that he was said to be nervous as a child, and would sometimes vomit before going to school. It was only then that I vividly recalled my night visit to him when he was eighteen months old. I had heard from his grandmother about his younger sister, adopted when he was about five, but he gave me an uncomprehending stare when I asked how they got on, then his "very well of course" seemed to bring his willingness to talk to me to an end. We parted with the decision that he would continue under the care of the psychiatrist.

But the old lady was not prepared to let the matter drop. Two weeks later, when she was in about her arthritis, she shook her head about Roy, and said that she understood a great deal more of what went on than his parents, but she couldn't interfere. Still, she was doing so to some effect, for her son, Roy's father made an appointment himself to discuss Roy with me. Very uncharacteristic!

Roy's father, in shiny office suit and round toed black shoes had a prevailing air of ownership of the business, rather than partnership with his more casual brother. Both deferred to their mother, as if she still had some control over them. Portly, short, owlish behind his spectacles, hesitant in speech, slow in thought and expression of feeling, his obsessive manner made even a simple query about a monthly account, an arduous undertaking. He was clearly a man more at ease with his receipts and estimates in his own office, than when asking for help in mine.

He blushed a little, and attempted a prim smile. He cleared his throat, but his voice piped, and broke. His uneasiness spoke of his lack of confidence in the competence of a man in his office.

"I don't know whether you will ... er ... agree with me. As a doctor I ... er ... expect you may know a bit more than me about this sort of thing. But in my layman's opinion,

Roy's troubles began with an incident when he was four ..."

I was surprised and pleased. I had not expected to find in him a congenial spirit. He continued with more confidence.

"We always intended having a second child, and when Roy was two and a half, my wife became pregnant again, but had a miscarriage. We decided to try again after a short while. Of course we were hoping for a little girl. When the baby was due Roy was mad with excitement. He was nearly five, and had seen a little girl born to my brother's wife ."

He choked a little. His round face began to look a bit squashed. The man wept, slightly.

"I'll cut it short ... the baby was stillborn ... we couldn't tell Roy, I thought he was too young, well I didn't know how to ... just brought the wife home two days later from hospital. He was waiting for us at the door, ran out to meet us .... watched us come out of the car by ourselves ... no baby .... I'll always remember this .... he said, 'Where's the baby, Dad, in the suitcase?'"

He smiled. His bland office exterior concealed the heart of a man and a father after all. He had re-created the drama mordantly enough for me to feel the pain of it, to picture the group at the front door without the baby, to compare my own experience of older children gazing in awe at the new baby. None of that for little Roy, aged five – just pain.

"Next year we adopted a little girl, Julie. But I don't think Roy ever got over it."

That was all he wanted me to know, and I thanked him and agreed to his request that I see Roy again. An appointment was made, but it was his father who came at the appointed hour, to say that Roy was ill at home, couldn't swallow and couldn't be persuaded to leave the house. I agreed to visit him there.

His mother showed me into a sitting room with comfortable arm chairs and television, a conventional suburban room, with french windows onto a garden, and there Roy sat mute and scared. It was his mother who told me that he complained of a sore throat. He didn't speak and as she had left us very quickly, the situation was bizarre. I examined him, and found nothing but his obvious anxiety, his throat was perfectly healthy. I asked him to call his mother back. I was surprised to realize that he couldn't. He was too paralyzed by fear to leave the room. This was reminiscent of the drama in the lay-by.

Before I left, I asked his mother if she remembered my visit twenty years earlier, the first and last time we had spoken to one another. She remembered it well and, told me, as we stood on the doorstep, of similar episodes in Roy's childhood. She then decided to arrange an appointment with me for herself.

Mrs Wood was a pleasant woman, in her mid forties, dark haired and homely. She was Italian by birth, but spoke with scarcely an accent. She met her husband after the war, and now expressed herself in English with greater fluency than he could.

Roy had frequent nightmares as an infant and toddler, she said, sometimes he would scream for hours on end. At first they called the doctor out, but later found that they could nurse him out of it themselves. He shared their bedroom until he was five and would not hear of parting from them at bedtime. When he started school, there had been screaming and struggling at the school gate. She took him to the Child Guidance Clinic at Great Ormond Street, every Tuesday for a year. This was the time of the miscarriage and the still birth. But even in the years before that, Roy would never be separated from them.

"They told us at the Clinic he was a 'worry guts'. We could never leave him with anyone, even his granny. If we brought him round to her house in the car and left him there so that we could go shopping on our own, before we turned round, he was already back in the driving seat waiting for us: he'd nip out of the house before we noticed and on no account stay without us. Sometimes he was so quiet and still we forgot he was there, other times he lay flat on the floor and screamed if we tried to move him. He never did well at school because he was always in a trance. The only thing he was ever interested in was cars, and now, he won't hardly go anywhere in a car, even his own."

She asked me what I thought they ought to do, they didn't like Roy drugged on the tablets, and in any case they didn't help. I repeated that talking and discussion was the method I favoured, to establish the continuity with his childhood separation anxieties. And did I think that he ought to come off the depression tablets? Yes, I agreed with them that it was an unpleasant idea for a young man to be on sedatives for years.

Roy recovered spontaneously from this attack: a few days later he waved to me insouciantly from the forecourt. His father rang later, they had told the psychiatrist that I suggested talking to Roy more, and he had replied, "Oh, the Dutch Uncle treatment? I don't think that will do much good!"

No decision was made, except to try to omit the tablets.

Soon grandmother's anxiety increased again, she began to suspect that she had some internal complaint that required hospital investigation. Arthritis and diverticulitis were discovered, which she considered bearable.

She regained her composure and became thoughtful about the approaching re-development of the area, and the demolition of the garage. Unlike her grandson she welcomed the opportunity to talk about herself and her feelings. The transport business linked her emotionally not only with her late husband but with her parents. They were Oxfordshire villagers who made the move to London in Edwardian times, before the First World War. Her father had left his father's smallholding and managed slowly to build up a connection with a horse and wagon, transporting goods to St Pancras and Oxford. Her mother had come to London to seek an alternative to domestic service in a country house. The couple met at the house of his older sister, an earlier immigrant to the city. Mrs Woods was only fourteen when her father died from tuberculosis. Her mother, who lived to be ninety, had been left with thirteen children, of whom she was the youngest.

She herself married at nineteen and with her husband established the garage, and passed it on to their two sons. But now they had decided to part. Roy and his father would buy a new garage in the suburbs. Her other son and his wife would find a village store in the West Country, and she would live in the flat over it. She thought that having lived over a business all these years she would find an ordinary house too quiet.

Some weeks later, Roy came in, again complaining of a sore throat, which in fact was perfectly healthy in appearance. He was once more on a full dose of anti-depressants and still unable to drive a car without his father in the passenger seat. He gazed at me uncomprehendingly. There was silence. I asked him if he wanted to try talking about it with me again. He said he would ask his father. His father agreed, but warned me that once his son had made up his mind nothing could shift him.

Roy's blankness, a sign of a vegetating imagination, of an emotional life whose low vitality was further subdued by sedation, was intimidating. I had seen his near psychotic states of confusion and felt the creepy impact of projections from his often disjointed mind. But no discussion could be sustained about his relationship with anyone, neither his father, mother, adopted sister, grandmother, cousin, or ex-fiancée.

He was puzzled and guilty about his intense separation anxieties but it was in the nature of his problem that in order to think about it, he would have to mobilise his imagination. But this implied my freedom to think whatever I wished, and this challenged his desire to control his environment, and of course his parents externally and internally.

He told me that his parents had planned a holiday by themselves, and confessed that he had managed to veto the idea.

We had a few exchanges of this nature:

"What I want to know is, why do my nerves affect what I love most, cars?"

"I think because cars are connected in your mind with the people that you love most, your parents. The problem was getting connected with your girl friend . . . ."

"That's rubbish."

"I think you have difficulty in thinking about unfamiliar ideas?"

"It's true that at school I used to sit in a trance, hearing the teacher's voice in the distance. And if they shouted at me I used to get worried. Your idea just seems silly to me, but if there is anything it it, it scares me because it means I might have another breakdown like in the lay-by. That's why I can't think of going without the tablets, I can't take the risk of going through that again."

"Courage would be needed . . . ."

"Point is I've never been interested in people, only cars.

54

Just now for example I'm going to sell an E-type Jag I've been working on, and buy a big American type. Money is a necessary evil, but I don't mind spending it, it seems so stupid that I have this thing about cars of all things!"

"Perhaps you could give some thought to this idea that the cars are connected with people that you love, and that there's a little boy in you that gets frightened when they go out of sight, and then you can't be sure where they are or what they're doing. After all cars have the advantage that they are always under your control."

"I'm sorry I just don't see it. Is there any point in us going on?"

That night I dreamed that I was disappointed in my hope of curing a young man of multiple sclerosis.

He failed the next weekly appointment, but came across the road to apologise half an hour later. When he failed to turn up the next time, there was no message until I happened to see him at the pumps, the next day. I had not mentioned to him that I would expect him to pay for any missed sessions. I suggested he would be more likely to remember to come if I charged him for them, as was my usual practice. A look of pain disturbed his blandness, and he staggered back, tripping on the plinth of the kiosk. He kept the next appointment.

He sat in silence, and I filled in the time with talk about how I thought cars were related to problems dating from his infancy about the fear of being separated from his parents. After a while, I asked him again to try to talk to me about what was going through his mind, and he eventually burst out with some passion, that I was making him feel angry by insisting on what sounded like rubbish to him. Still, he said he wished to continue, and we agreed to meet again in two weeks after the Easter holiday. He helpfully suggested that a Monday would be better as he would be able to remember the weekend difficulties more easily. As it happened, in the meantime, I thought it best to refuse a cheque proffered by his father on the grounds that it was preferable for Roy to conduct that business with me himself.

If this incident played a part in the succeeding drama, I am uncertain, but when Roy came for his session his mood was quite different. He sat down and said immediately that he felt better with the tablets, that without them he was quite unable to drive alone even for short distances. He had come to end the therapy there and then. I wanted to let him feel that I was not abandoning hope, and would not collude with a sudden departure.

We stayed together discussing various matters as they came to mind, mainly to do with economics. I mentioned the incident with the cheque offered by his father and he told me of his unease when owing or owed money. I linked it to emotional indebtedness, and how it might affect his ability to learn from other people, and his loss of interest in school lessons. He gave me to understand that he was making contact with the psychiatrist again and we parted on the understanding that he could return, should he wish to do so.

Then the stability of the locality came to an end. A compulsory purchase order was placed on the garage. Soon the forecourt, house and workshops were flattened by bulldozers and the site screened from view by corrugated iron sheets. Another order was expected shortly for the surgery premises. Only the pub would remain in place and continue as before.

Roy's uncle sold his share in Wood's Garage to his brother, and bought his grocery store in the West Country, taking the old lady with him. But Mrs Wood was restless so far away from London and returned, disconsolate, until a flat was found near Cyril and his family: they had found a garage on the outskirts of London and moved there.

The old lady travelled in to see me with a mild 'flu, but soon returned to her concern with her grandson.

"His father wants him to manage the garage, but it won't work. Roy's only happy if he spends the whole day in the workshop. He's a sick boy, he isn't capable of running a garage. Have you heard the latest development?"

I had heard nothing from the family since they moved out.

"He's made friends with a Canadian car mechanic. He says he is a qualified nurse and that he knows what's the matter with Roy and can cure him, it's so ridiculous. He's moved into the house, pays nothing for rent or keep, and they all think the world of him. He says he's a psychiatrist! He's no more of a psychiatrist than I am! D'you know he actually prevented my son from coming to collect me from the coast one weekend, because he said Roy couldn't stand being without them! I know what I think. I think he's a bad influence, but there's nothing I can do about it."

Roy too, kept turning up complaining of his throat from time to time during the following year. I learned that the male nurse did not last very long. Then visits from both grandmother and grandson ceased, and I heard no more of their story.

A passer-by would now have no hint of the geography of that locality as it was. They would have to consult one of those dusty picture post cards that sometimes survive, showing the streets as they used to be in bygone days. The traffic island and its vortex have gone. A supermarket now occupies the site of Wood's Garage, the house and the workshops. The surgery and the rest of the terrace came down and were replaced by a traffic round-about. The pub underwent a facelift and refurbishment, but has not managed to rid itself of its monolithic raffishness. The practice continues from premises on the new housing estate . . . .

5   That boy!

One morning, two clattering, chattering elderly ladies, tumbled over one another into the consulting room. With cries and sighs of relief, they dumped down their bulging shopping bags, and staked out a claim to much of the floor space. Even before they settled themselves into chairs, they began to recommend themselves as excellent trouble free patients. Also they had heard that I was likely to meet their need for a doctor who was above all clean. They were mother-in-law, and daughter-in-law, the two Mrs Cooks.

Seated to left and to right of me, they lobbed and volleyed words over my head, with the anticipation of seeded tennis players, and as they took the phrases from each other's lips, intercepted, rallied and smashed, I was obliged, like a spectator at Wimbledon, to turn my head from side to side, to follow the action.

"Old fashioned" was my first thought, "they are two astounding old fashioned eccentric strange ladies, who may give me much trouble." Mrs Edith Cook, seventy years old, sturdy and erect, in a substantial wool coat of dark grey, and time out of mind old lady's plain felt hat looked the more formidable. Grey eyes glimmered at me through brown spectacle frames: was that severity or a tight smile? For any expression more committed to light heartedness, it seemed there would be some machinery to adjust. The angle of her mandible, and the hair subjugated by braiding, spoke of feminity battened down and secured by discipline and muscularity.

Mrs Dora Cook, married to Edith's younger son Jim, and without children of her own, was more timid: smaller, rounder, mezzo-soprano to the other's contralto. She was agitated, clamorous, ready to submit, or to fly if snubbed. Through the flat lenses of her plain spectacles she peeped out as if from behind a curtain. She was decidedly hump-backed, the consequence of tuberculosis of the spine, in her adolescence. She had been treated as a long term hospital patient in pre-chemotherapy days, with enclosure in a plaster of Paris corset

59

and then strapped, so she said, to a steel frame. But today she wore, like her mother-in-law, a warm dark coat, with utilitarian buttons and a hat secured with a hat pin.

They wished to register as patients. Dr Craven, their previous doctor, had retired and been replaced. His successor had in some way offended them. They gave no details, but said they were sorry for his wife. Dr Craven had been a wonderful man, both as husband, father and doctor, and had been to them — they wished me to be clear about this — *"more of a friend than a doctor,"* I was to understand that this possibility of intimacy was also open to me, should I desire it. There was no delicacy in these initial courtesies, these ladies operated not so much with hints as with the dig of an elbow. Their tumultuous entry into the room was the first move in their anxious intention to make me an offer that I could not refuse. Old Dr. Craven was much in their minds as a medical ideal. They seemed to know all about his private life. They emphasized how clean he had been, and indeed how clean they found me. This other doctor fellow they accused of being dirty, but I wondered what exactly they meant, how they came to these conclusions, what enquiries they had made, and that perhaps — I didn't know really what they were talking about — they might after all find they had made a mistake about me. A quick glance round confirmed what I already knew — that my room was dusty in the corners and I was doubtful about the current state of my finger nails.

The atmosphere of the consultation was now calmer, as their excitement and anxiety and my suspicion calmed down. They were very knowledgeable about the district and its population. They seemed to have inside information about the local government's plans to redevelop the area, including their own street, and were sceptical about its competence. Old Mrs Cook had lived there for at least sixty years, and deplored the deterioration in housing and amenities that had taken place around her.

The medical business of the consultation was dispatched quickly, they each required a monthly prescription of laxatives and arthritic tablets. Dora also required ointment for mild psoriasis, and some bland cream for the genital area, which had a tendency to become sore, examination declined.

We seemed to have many mutual acquaintances: one or two

families who were my patients were their distant relatives, many of their neighbours seemed to confide their family and medical problems to them. I began to sense that they were an important piece in the jigsaw of local life. This was an experience I had noticed occasionally: after some years of visiting homes in a certain street, I would take on a family who lived in a house I had often passed, and discover they had all along been significant to the life of the street, and they knew a surprising amount about me.

How often, passing a couple of people, pausing for a chat in the street, I overheard them talking about their illnesses and what the doctor said. (When I remembered about this it sometimes had a modulating effect on what in fact I did say in the consultation.) Mrs Cook senior, whom I could now discern had a certain queenly and proprietary air in relation to Forest Road where she lived, and to outlying territories, no doubt participated in many such conversations. In fact she confided as we went on talking, that she felt some of the people we both knew about would be better off if they were not so weak willed, and took a stronger line not only with themselves but with their families.

I was not being made to work. I was being charmed, entertained. I sat back and enjoyed their company, in no hurry for them to go. We might have continued much longer but for other patients waiting, and I reluctantly stood up to put them in mind of departure, and helped them to gather together their shopping. They delayed their exit by remarking once again on how strongly I put them in mind of old Dr Craven — just like him apparently — and then they suddenly recollected how fond he had been of their scones and enquired whether I also liked home made cake and if so would I have any objection if on their next visit they brought a little something along?

Thereafter they called once a month, to renew their prescriptions: ointments and tablets for them, home baked scones and cake for me. I had inherited their friendship with old Dr. Craven.

In the years ahead we grew fond of one another, and I found it hard to recapture that initial impression of absurd eccentricity or the anxiety that they would be troublesome to me. While their symbiosis was absolute, and they thought and acted with uncanny unity, that antique sobriety concealed geniality of manic force. Intolerant of weakness in themselves, or their neighbours, yet they used their superiority in intelligence, energy and wealth, to assist them if they could.

They lived in Forest Road, in the network of little streets, off the main road. This street abutted at its farther end onto a footpath which ran by the ancient parish church and its peaceful grounds, where old plane trees provided shade for time-worn graves. At the other end, where it met the high road, all was noise and traffic and hustle. From the Cooks' house near the footpath, could be seen the first new dwellings of the housing estate that would in a few more years, engulf the whole locality. They hoped they would have gone by then to a cottage by the sea. They had already bought it and visited there two or three times a year. They were waiting for Dora's husband's retirement, still some ten years ahead.

The older Cooks had lived there since their marriage, and it was cleaned, dusted and swept with rigour, and preserved, like the ladies themselves, in a style of indeterminate age. The floral wall paper, heavy curtains and nets, the overstuffed arm chairs, that took up too much space, the polished dining table and upholstered seats of the dining chairs, came from affluence beyond their neighbours'.

They were sensitive to the problems of the less fortunate in that declining locality, but were frustrated by the difficulty of doing much other than offering moral support. Indignation with the immutability of the social and economic problems that surrounded them, often expressed itself as exasperation with the passivity of others in those streets less energetic and hopeful than themselves. But from their strategic position at the head of Forest Road, they kept an eye on the welfare of their indigenous neighbours and their children. I was in one or other of that network of streets visiting, nearly every day. Home visits were frequent there, but it was a human place, animated with homely activities, as the inhabitants came and went about their business and the children played in the street. A fishmonger traded from a handcart, and a small time bookmaker took bets in a doorway, before betting shops were legal. The shops on the High Road were only a step away, someone was always coming or going, children shouted, the elderly sunned themselves, dogs sniffed around, livelier cats prowled after the sparrows and pigeons fluttered from the roof tops to peck at crumbs.

This triangular territory between the railway line and the parish church, was divided up by short straight streets. The terraced houses gave directly onto the pavements at the front, and had small gardens at the back. They were now more than a hundred years old. Many were divided between two families, with outside toilets and no bathroom. The Council planners had decided against refurbishing, demolition was the word, and re-development. Twenty years later when the shoddy dwellings of the housing estate and the new slums of the point blocks began to deteriorate, they realised they had made a mistake.

Meanwhile, some of the houses were occupied by inhabitants whose parents had given birth to them there, sixty or seventy years ago. Here and there an old widower struggled on without his wife; widows kept up the neatness of their parlours, and looked for a visit from their grandchildren from the suburbs. Empty flats were taken over by immigrants, Irish and West Indian. A simple minded Jewish woman had somehow got left behind, from an earlier wave of immigration.

My first call to their terrace house had been for the elder Mr Cook. Dora's husband — Edith's son — was often spoken of, but not the old man who completed the household. On this first visit, I was shown upstairs, to a dimly lit bedroom where Edith's husband was largely concealed by a heavy eiderdown. Access was difficult to his side of the conjugal bed, against the wall, and an oversized chest of drawers and wardrobe was in the way, on the other. He looked ancient, an old man with grey moustache and grizzled cheeks, who smiled wanly as I reached over the corner of the furniture to take his pulse. He apologised for, rather than complained of, chest pain. Both ladies and Jim who had crowded in behind me, thought that if it was a heart attack he would be best in hospital. The diagnosis was confirmed there, but he died after a few days, aged seventy five. I had thought he was older.

He was mourned, as he had lived in that household, unob-trusively. I cannot remember much fuss being made about his going. They liked cleanliness and hygiene in death as in life, and the old man, the only silent member of the quartet, went quietly.

With time, the complexities of their family history were confided to me. Edith Cook met all blows from fate with good temper, irritation was reserved for weakness in others, she had no time for neighbours or relatives who cowered in adversity.

When Doris was sixteen, they told me, she was found by her future mother-in-law, at work with bent back behind the counter of a local wet fish shop. "Abandoned by her family," they said. I was unable to penetrate beyond this point in her history. Mrs Cook senior took pity on her, gave her lodging, and henceforth presided over her health and welfare.

The foundling developed an attachment to her saviour, passionate and tenacious. Mrs Cook had two sonss, but no daughters, and the two became so inextricably needful of each other, that their identities merged, their thoughts synchronized, their talk blended in harmony, and parted in counterpoint. Doris married Jim, the younger son, and was never far from her benefactress' side. Jim, burly, tall, red faced and a practical man about the house, held down an excellent job as clerk of works to a large firm. But in matters of health he was as nervous as a kitten. Now he had two ladies to support, he worried endlessly.

Some years after the death of her husband, I answered an urgent call to Edith, who was haemorrhaging. Later, I visited her in hospital as she recovered from a resection of the bowel for cancer. Idealisation of medical powers accelerated, in response to the need for hope. My presence at her bedside, when she knew that she would have a colostomy confirmed her opinion of my worthiness to sit with Dr Craven in their pantheon of well scrubbed physicians.

Not only did they defer to my opinions, but more home made cake was pressed on me with cups of tea on my visits, and sent home with me for my family. At Easter, large fruit and cream cakes, scones, puddings and pastry reached gourmandising proportions; at Christmas there were several boxes packed with brandy soaked Christmas puddings "cut and come again" fruit cake, mince pies, apple tarts, sponge cake iced with orange and pink sugar, and stuffed with whipped cream, together with chocolates, sweets, trinkets and toys for the children.

As the Cook ladies took an interest in the welfare of their neighbours, should one of them fall ill (and if they were my patients,) I would feel an enhanced responsibility. I was anxious that my clean reputation should not tarnish.

Across the road at number 28, in an upstairs flat conversion of a terrace house, lived a retired engine driver, in the care of his unmarried daughter. He was a tall dignified man of eighty, who looked like Sir Adrian Boult. The care and propriety with which he was serviced by his daughter was praised by the Cook ladies. In contrast, and to my distress, they remained aloof and disinterested in Mr Lloyd. He was a Welshman, who had sunk into despair since the death of his wife ten years earlier. I had attended her in her last months in the upstairs back bedroom, where she died of cancer. He was dirty and ill fed, living off loaves of bread and canned milk, increasingly alcoholic and paranoid. I had a tenuous exemption from his suspicions, and I liked to listen to his musical voice, as he described his life as a young man. He had been a mining engineer, and had travelled extensively in South America, but now in his soiled shirt and greasy suit, slumped on a battered wooden chair at the kitchen table, in the dismal back living room, that had seen no decoration for over a decade, he was disenfranchised from the ladies' concern, because "*he had let himself go*".

The ladies did worry about the son of their nephew who lived next door. Simon came into the world with an imperforate anus. This was of course speedily corrected surgically, but imperfect sphincter control marred his life. He was also an accident prone juvenile deliquent, but the connection with his handicap was unclear. The Cooks referred to him as "that boy!". Over tea and a slice of cake in the back parlour, I would be told the latest news of him:

"That boy! We just can't understand him. Doctor, I blame his parents. They're not firm enough with him, and he's ..."

"... in trouble again," said Dora, "cut his head open, breaking into an empty house with that gang of ruffians and ...."

"... mind you, I'll say this, he's never played like other

65

children, always broke his toys, straight off, even when he was a tot. Can you imagine, parents buying a boy like that an airgun? . . . ."

" . . . makes us think they've less sense than him . . . ."

"D'you know what I'd do if I was his father? I'd give him a damn good hiding, Cecil's soft with him."

I knew his parents well, they were unsophisticated, timid and confused, but they had a perfectly normal elder daughter, and had reason to feel that it was not "all their fault". Five years ago, I had told them that I thought he needed psychological help, but he was ten before they agreed to take him to a child guidance clinic, concerned by the frequent minor accidents he inflicted on himself. He had fractured his wrist and ankle, cut himself innumerable times, and with his harassed mother, was a familiar at the practice. He had undergone a remarkable amount of surgery for one so young — the repair to his anus at birth, an undescended testicle operation, and numerous other minor procedures.

The child psychiatrist agreed that he was a disturbed little fellow, and that in the diagnositic sessions he expressed dislike of both his mother and his father. Clearly he also disliked the chief victim of the psychopathic element in his personality — himself. But his baffled and guilt ridden parents had no concept of psychotherapy, and the opportunity for help of that kind was missed. As a young adult he was imprisoned more than once for drug offences, and nearly died from hepatitis from a dirty needle.

Another problem for the Cooks was a distant relative, a thirty year old bachelor, who lived at home with his parents, a few streets away. He had a depressive breakdown, refused to go to work, was unable to use public transport, and spent his days sitting at home ruminating on the meaninglessness of his existence. In contrast to the Cooks, he had little faith in me or any other doctor, found waiting rooms intolerable, and a referral to the hospital psychiatrist foundered on his inability to travel or to wait.

After some occasional discussions, over two or three years, we discovered that the problem was related to his envy of a younger brother, who had married and started a family. With some work on this, he improved considerably, and the ladies were confirmed in their pride of possession of me. Indeed there was much cosy mutual admiration, and I took medical students there, on the pretext of a routine visit, to demonstrate a good doctor-patient relationship, and to share their excellent home made cream sponge.

Across the road from them lived Mrs O'Brien, who was similar to them only in two respects, the impact of a first excited meeting, and a subsequent capacity to fascinate me. But her character and way of life were so antipodean to theirs, that although I visited and was fond of both, and they all lived in the same street, they might have been on different planets. I wished that I could have introduced them to each other, and made them friends.

Mrs O'Brien was a widowed Irish lady of about sixty, when I first met her. She had sent for me to attend her privately at her little terrace house. She received me in a state of considerable sexual excitement. A provocative decolletage, droll coyness, vague but melodramatic hypochondria, and stage Irish eloquence, hypnotised me at once. A small neat, comely body, with untidy grey hair, she was animated by the persistence of little girl flirtatiousness into her early old age. I found nothing wrong with her, other than her inappropriate ardour of expression and anxiety. She soon registered as a National Health Service patient, but continued always to press pound notes into my hand.

She had a lodger with whom she denied co-habiting, to some extent. She was involved in an indeterminate financial and legal struggle over a business of some kind she had retired from before moving into the area. She had a rich son, and two daughters, one of whom could be relied on, and one who was ill herself and could not.

She suffered from palpitations and panic attacks of histrionic proportions. Her complex hypochondriacal anxieties were part of a nervous disposition, three parts depression to two parts of hypomania. She was ambivalent towards everyone, including of course myself. She idealised, and denigrated, in successive breaths. Having told me what a wonderful doctor I was, she would tell me that her son had said "bugger Dr Sanders!" She could not see me at home, or at the surgery without distributing small presents: fruit and chocolate for the receptionists, a folding umbrella, a book of rabbinical sermons, slippers for my wife, groceries, drink. It was easier and pleasanter to accept than to refuse these offerings, which she pressed on all who served her, plumbers, ambulance men, decorators, the priest . . . .

Bill Franks, her lodger, insisted on private patient status from the start, and stuck to it. He was sixty four inches tall, but weighed eighteen stone. Rough and rubicund in appearance, he would come through the consulting room door, cautiously, a travel stained car coat open over a baggy pullover. I think he worried that his liaison with Mrs O'Brien, interfered with my willingness to have him in the room. In this he confused me with her family, who found her evasiveness about him fuelled their exasperation.

His smoker's wheezy chest often required antibiotic support. Perhaps to economise in breath he kept his cockney speech to a minimum and always to the point, unlike his landlady. An arthritic hip gave him a rolling gait but his bluff sea-faring taciturnity served only to navigate a small battered van the length and breadth of southern England.

He was hurt when my senior partner refused to take him as a private patient. Bill deduced it was because he did not look financially sound, for when he came to me, on the rebound, he pulled a soiled but fat wad of ten pound notes from the hip pocket of his ample trousers, and told me he earned hundreds of pounds, cash down, transporting goods, night and day, cross country, in his van. I found him absolutely resistant to weight loss, although he desired this more than anything. He was uncommunicative about his relationship to Mrs O'Brien or about anything else. When he died suddenly of a heart attack, in his van, far from home, Mrs O'Brien was hysterical.

I made a note once, as near as I could remember, of Mrs O'Brien's confusing but hypnotic rhetoric. I did this to calm myself when I returned from an urgent call from a frightened neighbour, who thought she might be terribly ill:

"Oh, Doctor, thank God you've come God bless us and save us I didn't think I'd live another minute the central heating exploded there's water all over the place the men came and didn't do a thing and sent me a bill for eight pounds I went to

my Donald's for the weekend and just had five pounds on me
I went into their little bedroom and put my little case on the
shelf and his wife said to me what do you think you're doing
and I said only putting my little case on the shelf and she said
you mustn't do that and emptied my case into a drawer and
took it away well I had five pounds on me I gave ten shillings
each to the little girls for their bazaar and I rang up a cab
driver such a nice man and I said how much will you charge
to take me back home he's a lovely man he said three pounds
ten I said how long will it take you I said and he said twenty
five minutes so I packed my things and I left without saying
anything to anyone and when his wife found I'd gone she was
that angry she rang my Mary although I'm from peasant
stock myself they think they are way above us and my Mary
said to her you can go to hell and my brother can go to hell
and your family can go to hell and get off my bloody
telephone oh Doctor when I got back here there were mice in
my sitting room my kitchen is so clean I have never ever had
anything like that before my Kathleen started to chase them
around and I said don't kill them don't kill them I can't stand
that my Kathleen's husband Arnold Price he could come here
and fix my central heating but he doesn't bother he didn't like
my Bill none of them liked my Bill I'll never be the same now
that Bill's gone I'm nobody now my Donald said to me I was
living in sin with Bill I said to him I've no sins I've been to
confession I've called a priest I can't get to mass now the
priest comes to me and I give him a pound well thanks for
coming and listening to me thank Jesus and Mary I feel a
little better I'm saving up my money and when it comes to
Christmas I'm going to buy you and that other lovely doctor
some whisky goodbye now, goodbye."

The Cook family could not do with this kind of hysteria and
took no notice of poor Mrs O'Brien, who eventually went off to
live with her Mary.

Dora Cook's husband Jim was a hesitant talker and in any
case, not often called upon to speak by the ladies, but he was a
virtuoso of property repair and home maintenance. He won
praise as an unparalleled son and husband — idealized, the
clean one — and his unblemished record contrasted with the

bad character of his elder brother Jack, a successful business man, of whose lavish life style, large country house, and fast cars they very much disapproved.

The true cause of their distress was that after his wife deserted him, Jack asked his family to take care of Brian, his two year old son, of whom he had the custody. Dora and Jim, being childless, gladly agreed to foster and later adopt him, and he was brought up thereafter in the care of the ladies and Uncle Jim of Forest Road. But his father was waiting for him, had plans for his future. At seventeen Brian found that a place was reserved for him in his father's business, and he stepped into ready-made affluence. Brian did his best with his divided loyalties but conflict about whose son he was, remained unresolved. He visited Forest Road from time to time, where photographs of the grandchildren were exhibited, and the ladies were proud of his success. I was told of a magnificent house built by the firm for Brian and his young family, and of its sale at an enormous profit, but their satisfaction at Brian's happiness and wordly success was marred by an ache of heartbreak, and the responsibility for it was laid on Jack.

Jim, his stay-at-home younger brother, proficient man about the house, burly and pink cheeked, was easily put out by medical problems, and this childlike timorousness rendered him worse than useless when the ladies were ill. Usually it was possible to calm his trusting nature with a promise of speedy recovery, and he could then escape back to practical jobs at work and at home. In his chosen field, he was, according to his womenfolk, a prodigy, a prototype of excellence, whose qualities shone the more resplendent, because of his older brother's surrender of eternal values to vulgar materialism and success in business. These praises caused Jim's pink cheeks to glow with healthy pride, in the satisfaction of being needed, and of acknowledged usefulness. It was the basis of his domestic felicity.

I think it unlikely that Dora and Jim ever consummated their marriage. Dora asked me to examine her once, many years after I first met her. She had told me about her prolapsed uterus, but I was not expecting to find that it protruded so far. She declined to submit herself to the knife, and continued as before to use copious amounts of cream and ointment to protect herself from soreness.

Her mother-in-law took a sympathetic though detached view of Dora's morbidity, which induced in her a childlike submissiveness. Perhaps it was those years of hospital life strapped to a frame, which induced her to yield herself up medically, rather than conjugally. I had examined her spine, at her invitation, on an earlier occasion. She went ahead to her bedroom to undress, and called me when she was ready. I found her lying in the middle of the double bed naked, with the bed coverings folded to the foot of the bed.

In that little girl-like willing exhibition of her naked body, in her case sadly deformed by the twisted angularity of her spine, I was reminded of on an elderly lady who, left to the last in the waiting room, calmly took off all her clothes and sat naked until she was called: this heralded the relapse of her schizophrenia.

One day old Mrs Cook noticed she was breathless, and her ankles were swollen. She was tipping over into heart failure, and was rescued with diuretics and digitalis. But the idea of her mother-in-law's mortality was ominous for Doris. She reacted within three weeks by becoming so pale and short of breath herself, that the possibility of acute leukaemia came to mind. The blood count showed only simple iron deficiency anaemia, and this in spite of iron therapy, was almost immediately complicated .... by heart failure. She required exactly the same prescription of diuretic and digitalis tablets now as her analogue: the affinity was sustained.

A year later old Mrs Cook suffered a heart attack, and was admitted to hospital. Her son and his wife behaved with admirable calmness this time, and took her back home to nurse with efficient solicitude. They were helped in this, as they had been for some years with the colostomy, by an incomparable District Nurse, who I first met when I came to the practice. She was now semi-retired, but maintained her bonny maternal attractiveness and when she was in attendance the battle was half won, without any doctor's assistance. Her calmness, competence and experience, were exemplary, and when she retired, the area was depleted. She was quite unnecessarily bashful about her excellent consort, and the fact of being unmarried led to a few embarrassing moments, simply because of her reluctance to acknowledge his presence, as he waited in his car outside a patient's house. She had three daughters from a previous marriage, one of whom died in young motherhood, but I never heard why she did not remarry.

Finally, Mrs Cook senior, was carried off by her third coronary thrombosis, at the age of eighty. The others took it without any major show of grief. They felt, they said, that a most unusual and excellent person had left them, and they now had to make the best of their lives together. They kept her embalmed in the front parlor waxed and rouged for five days and showed me a letter from an old friend, who wrote that she would plant a rose bush in her garden in her memory and would have a chat with it now and again.

The demolition of the little streets and terrace houses now accelerated, obliging the inhabitants to disperse, some to old age homes, some to distant suburbs, some to new towns. Before long the new estate would take shape, blocks of flats with expensive central heating, and modern kitchens — and flat roofs that let in the rain and in fifteen years would require to be replaced with old fashioned sloping ones.

Jim and Dora wasted no more time, and retired to the seaside cottage as they had long planned. We continued to exchange Christmas cards to the end of their lives, but never met again.

6   Evacuee

Mrs Rogers wanted an opinion on what she should do about her husband, who was not a patient of the practice.

Three months ago, she said, his body had been found slumped half out of his car, on a south coast beach. He had been taken to the nearest hospital, treated for drug overdose, and three days later, sent back to London. He was now attending a local out-patient clinic, taking anti-depressants. She had no idea what would happen to him or to their marriage. He preferred not to come home, he was staying with his brother.

Mrs Rogers was in her forties, pretty, radiating discreet sexuality. I liked to see her, but was apprehensive of her turquoise eyes, wide and wondering beneath plucked brows: the charm of her melting glance distracted attention from whatever it was she wanted. Once her children's illnesses were over, she rarely came to see me about anything other than her breasts, which formed worrying little lumps from time to time.

She was a receptionist at an expensive hotel, and was required professionally to be glamorous in a prudent way. In the intimacy of the consulting room, the impact tended to the excessive. Her beauty was designed to dazzle from behind a protective barrier, a desk or a counter, to smooth the way for transactions with strangers. In the consulting room her unpretentious self, a worried mother and housewife, contended with her commercial persona.

I had in the past, given some support to a depressed friend of hers. The outcome of that led her to think I might help her husband. I agreed to meet him: he came alone at the appointed time, cautious, polite, in a dark grey suit, his wife's age. Traces of adolescent comeliness clung to his good-looking profile, his trimmed chestnut hair. His clear brow, frank brown eyes, and clean pale cheeks, were under-pinned by a strong jaw line and a determined, pointed chin. These latter helped to discount a suggestion of androgynous ambiguity. He looked unhappy, but not desperate, and seemed capable of good humour.

He had come, he said calmly, and his voice was pleasantly, quietly, resonant – not from the throat, but from the chest he had come for a second opinion. He was at present in the care of the psychiatrist at a general hospital in the neighborhood. As he was not improving, there was a proposal to admit him to the psychiatric ward. He had no idea what to do with himself but preferred not to return to live with his wife and the children.

The truth was — it came without unseemly embarrassment — that he had been having an affair with a girl. He presumed that was why he tried to kill himself, because he had behaved so stupidly, and because of the guilt. The whole affair had not been serious and was now quite irrelevant. His wife was frightened about what had happened, but still seemed to care for him, saw it as a breakdown, and was ready to forgive him. But he was not sure, felt confused and for the moment thought it was best to stay with his brother.

He had no job now, was disconnected from family and work, and in a strange way from perturbation, as he enquired whether, assuming it was worth the effort, I might have any idea how to save his life? If there was such an option, and his wife seemed to think there was, he was prepared to hear about it. But three months had passed, and he was no wiser now than on the day he had taken the overdose in his car on the beach.

Diffidently, but fluently, in that quietly resonant voice, he gave me more details. The incident with the girl had been trivial. He had decided to try a new office job outside London, met a girl down there, a secretary:

"I took her out for the first time just before Christmas. December 20 as a matter of fact. Nothing very serious: loneliness down there away from home, and she was friendly, a nice girl. Really there was nothing more to it. Just stupid."

His suicide attempt was six weeks later.

I asked some routine questions, for example about his parents. Astonishingly, he began with the fact that his father had died at the identical seaside resort, on the same date that he had just mentioned, twelve months before.

I felt this was ghoulish. My skin tingled. The same place, the same date a year earlier? Was all this business about the guilt and the infidelity and going to work at this seaside town, not the point? Had anyone commented to him on this stupefying . . . . fact? I could not say "coincidence." That would be mealy-mouthed.

He looked at me blankly. No, why?

I was surprised that this intelligent, calm, comely man, telling his story easily, from the chair at the right hand side of the desk, who wanted another opinion from me, and who was now about to have it, did not seem to share my astonishment. It was naive of me to expect enthusiasm, his mind was dulled by months of despair, but the difference between my agitation and his impassivity hurt. He was not even mildly interested, while I was awash with curiosity. His calm handsome face, his articulate speech, concealed the state of his imagination. It was weak.

Other facts were told. Twenty years ago, when he and his wife were first married, he moved in to live with her and her parents. Soon after, her mother went away with her lover. The three of them, Mrs Rogers and her two men, father and husband, could not find a way to live with this awkward arrangement. Mr Rogers and his father-in-law quarrelled. After a few months, his wife's conflict of loyalty unresolved, Mr Rogers moved out.

Eight months later he came back. Two sons were born with an interval of four years between them. When the youngest child was two years old, Mrs Rogers' mother's lover was killed in a traffic accident. Crushed and weeping, she too, came back, and was taken in.

We had been talking for an hour, and I was disturbed by the turbulence he did not feel. The story was incomplete and I suggested we continue on another occasion. He agreed, with a pleasant smile which showed he was sure no good would come of it.

I was powerfully affected by this interview. I felt upset about this gentle melancholy but indifferent man, who had been found dying in his car on a lonely beach, and did not know what to do next. He seemed to regret still being around, and submitted to discussion not because he was interested, or hopeful, but because his wife — like me — seemed to be upset. He did at least feel for her, he could observe that there was something that seemed to bother her, and he certainly felt that he owed her some redress. But was not the best thing to clear out of her life and allow her to bring up the children, without the complication of his misery?

But then his wife too was an enigma, with her obsessive fear of cancer of the breast. A few minutes conversation and a brief examination had always been enough to give her temporary relief. I wondered if I was so disturbed, because of her – the combination of beauty and cancerphobia jangled. The latter was an unconscious death warrant issued for someone. Perhaps her husband?

At the second consultation, I heard of matters no less disturbing, and ignominious: again hopelessness showed through placidity, and inappropriate gentility. He wanted to clarify an important point from our first meeting. His mother-in-law's lover had been his close friend, introduced into the family by himself, and of his own age. Naturally he had felt in some way responsible. This affair between his friend and his mother-in-law had confused them all. There was a mystery about the fatal car accident: no other car had been involved, no-one else was hurt, the car was just found off the motorway, on its side, and on fire.

When his mother-in-law returned to her husband, she spent many days in bed, eating nothing, weeping, overcome with guilt. Then the whole matter was smoothed over, and the marriage continued as before.

The feeling of ghostly affinity with his own suicide attempt in a car made my flesh creep again.

Meanwhile, Mr Rogers' own mother and father retired, and settled in the seaside town. He mentioned that after his father and mother left London, his own health began to deteriorate, and again pained me with his inability to hear the clamor from his inner life, his dependent affectionate child self suffering from their absence. Within twelve months of their move he had fallen and broken his leg, soon to be followed by a severe attack of shingles, around his abdomen.

Then came his father's death, forty eight hours after a heart attack. The date was 20 December.

I was silent, I could think of nothing useful to say, while he had melted a little and had become confiding. Part of his problem, he said, was that he found it very difficult to settle into employment. His trade was electronics, he was competent, with a proper pride in his ability, but a dispute would blow up between him and management, and he would find himself out of work, and out of place in a dole queue, feeling a fool, a skilled middle-aged man, with a family, lining up for social security. The truth was, he said, and he smiled a strange empty smile, that he had been sacked from one job, because he had gone without permission to attend his father's funeral.

Now that he was thinking, following a train of thought, waking up, I began to hope again that he would understand why I was so astonished that he had not linked his depression to his father's death. He went on: in despair and confused, after his dismissal, he decided on the spur of the moment to take a job as a postman. Then came a skin cancer under his left eye needing surgery and radiotherapy. Dispirited and hopeless, he collected some tablets from his GP and went off to try his luck at the seaside, where he lodged with his widowed mother.

The rest was simple, according to him. He flirted with the girl in the office, who no doubt found his charming manners and deceptive air of maturity irresistible; then having convinced himself of the absurdity of his existence, and the futility of the affair, he swallowed enough tablets and whisky to kill himself. His unconscious body was spotted by an evening stroller, exercising his dog on the beach.

He came to the end of the story and stopped abruptly: he closed the book. My interest in what happened next — or might happen — was for the moment unwelcome, an infringement of privacy. His contact with his inner life was spasmodic, his resonant voice promised deep soundings of his emotional life — then he was beached on the shallows. Hopefulness had stirred, but having lost it once, he was suspicious of an offer of its return.

I learned, eventually, that he had been separated from his parents for three years when he was eleven, in September 1939. The Government had decided to evacuate children from cities and the danger of Hitler's bombers, although the children may well have preferred to perish with their parents than survive without them. Confused parents found it impossible to refuse measures for their children's safety. He grew to adolescence, with the adult world too pre-occupied to notice that he was catastrophically affected by the separation from his mother and father, whom it was logical to assume might be killed without being seen again. He disappeared from his parents' sight, a North London Icarus, who fell unobserved, as in Auden's *Musee des beaux Arts*:

> 'About suffering they were never wrong,
> The Old Masters ....
> In Brueghel's *Icarus*, for instance, how everything turns away
> Quite leisurely from the disaster; the ploughman may
> Have heard the splash, the forsaken cry,
> But for him it was not an important failure; the sun shone
> As it had to on the white legs disappearing into the green
> Water; and the expensive delicate ship that must have seen
> Something amazing, a boy falling out of the sky,
> Had somewhere to get to and sailed calmly on.'

Mr Rogers the man, sat by the desk, baffled and disinterested. An unpleasant ironic smile which tried to settle on his even features, was displaced by a look of unhappiness when I asked about his evacuation. The atmosphere charged with passion as he talked.

He and his older sister were sent in a school party to the Midlands. He became ill with eczema soon after he arrived at his foster parents' house. The itchy weeping rash, erupted on his trunk and limbs, too severe to manage at home: he was transferred to the local hospital. When he came out, he found he had lost his place in the grammar school and allocated to an inferior one. This was devastating: his grammar school scholarship had been the most exciting thing in his life. His parents had been proud of him, the only one in his family of low waged workers ever to win a place in the sun, and one of only two boys from his street corner primary school to do so. What went amiss he was unable to tell me. Perhaps it was a clerical error, or they thought he was not robust enough for the tougher curriculum, but he never made his way back. His elder sister, two years his senior, who wept without stopping for three weeks, was sent home. It was three years before he returned, a dispirited fourteen year old.

Back in London after the war, he had left school at fifteen and was apprenticed to an engineering firm, before his two years of National Service in the RAF. Home again with his parents, he changed jobs several times before he found a post that suited him. He gradually learned the job, earned promotion, worked his way up. He married soon after, and moved in with his in-laws. Then came the curious events he had already explained to me.

Absorbed in this review of his early life, recalling the soreness, he came back to the present moment, in confusion. Once again he closed his mind down. He saw that I had been attending closely to his account, maybe I read in it something to his disadvantage:

"What are you getting at?" he asked blankly.

I gave him some idea of what was in my mind, that he was suffering from hopelessness revived by the death of his father, but with a painful precedent thirty years earlier when he was sent away from home.

The consultation had become a bore to him, and anyway it was time to stop. I offered him a further appointment, he protested that he couldn't see the point, but would come.

That evening I looked at some letters written home, and kept, from the time of my own evacuation. I was away for three months, not three years, but the separation had been an extraordinary experience. Early in September 1939, a few days after the declaration of war, my school assembled at the railway station by class. Gas masks had been issued in small brown cardboard boxes, which were suspended by string from our shoulders. Like my patient, I had just changed from primary to grammar school, and most of my companions were strangers.

A billet for my older brother and myself had been found in a country town. The foster parents were kind people, but from the time of our arrival I was accompanied by a mental cloud wherever I went. The letters home varied between unconvincing jokiness through depression to persecution. Preserved in them is the indignation of fifty years ago. Luckily we returned home in time for Christmas.

In short, I had a trenchant identification with my patient: a boy of eleven, a hundred miles from home, amongst strangers. At the wrong school, left behind by his sister, his weeping,

79

itching and scaling skin I understood as an eloquent sign of inner torment.

But the time when he and I could talk freely had passed. He was uneasy with my continued interest, which was not the same as his original concept of "another opinion". He was twenty minutes late next time, and silent. Curt in reply to my efforts, he merely said he felt "out in space" and lacked confidence in himself. His wife was unable to bear him in this depressed mood, and refused to have him home. As a matter of fact, he said, he had been feeling a little better, and had asked her about it, but she had sent him back to his relatives, with a couple of extra suitcases of clothes.

He had no more to say: the last half hour of this session had been hard to endure. It had been pervaded by sulky silence, by hopelessness, and suspicion of the ethics of my actions. As we contemplated one another, I struggled with the thought, implanted in me by his surliness, and fed by my own anxiety that I was in the grip of an irrelevant identification, that I was absurd to embark, simply through egoism, on a questionable course of treatment for a dangerous illness. He, in neat suit and tie, tasteful socks and polished shoes, did his polite best to prevent his symmetrical good looks from expressing scorn for the faint hope that something might come of these encounters. But he did say (didn't he?), that he had been feeling a little better.

But this was an ephemera, as if of no substantial relevance to our meeting with one another. By the end of the session I had almost forgotten the distinct *frisson* of relief it gave me, before it succumbed to the dismal news that his wife had sent him away. Behind the mask of cosmetic art, there was pain in her pretty eyes. No, she was not one to bear depression, but she had sought help for him, and I knew that she was on our side.

He failed the next appointment, but phoned a few days later, and came again. Hope had returned. After a bad week with suicide on his mind again, his wife had come to fetch him home.

He had no job, and wouldn't apply for one because a refusal would be humiliating. He was morose and irritating. What was wrong with him? He was hard to bear. Now he wanted to come regularly, but had little to say that was not boring or depressing. He had been for another job, but was worried by a pain in his

80

chest. A link with his father's sudden death from coronary thrombosis? He couldn't see that. He had never been easy with his father, who said he was too ambitious. He could not, would not see any link, or even anything interesting in a connection between the death of his father, and his own suicide attempt on its anniversary, a year later, in the same distant town.

He started work, but it was not right. He felt he had deceived his employers: he was a fraud, he'd tricked them, he was incompetent. Yes, he had the qualifications, but he got jobs because he could talk well, and the competition was poor. He had always felt this at home, with his parents and his sister. That grammar school scholarship was a case in point, he hadn't been able to keep up to the required standard.

> "My sister? She is a mistress at hiding her emotions. She felt father's loss deeply but didn't show it too much. What? Yes, she certainly showed her emotions when we were evacuated ..."

Now that he was back with his wife, and working, his only complaint was lack of confidence. I was due for a holiday, and told him about it, a month ahead. He had registered with the practice, and we had been meeting weekly for two months. The "second opinion" had got under way as psychotherapy, and I wanted to prepare him for the interruption. I mentioned his sister who had been able to express her emotions, and how their parents responded to that, when they were evacuated. This had not carried through with him, eczema then, shingles and skin cancer after his father's death, his abrupt abandoning of his identity for that of a postman, (his father had been a milkman) all spoke a language without words about his anguish.

He heard me, was not unfriendly but remained sceptical. He was grateful for the improvement, but the background to his depressive illness interested him less and less: even as I spoke to him about the link with his childhood, the years of separation, the death of his father, their meaning evaporated: interesting perhaps to those who found that sort of thing interesting, which he did not. But he returned the following week with something he did want to discuss. His eczema was back, his fingers blistered and peeled, for the first time since he was fifteen.

When we resumed on my return, three weeks later the talk

was of headaches and of eczema. This had some of his own personality, a type of restrained blistering like his scorn, rather than the weeping of his sister. He was impatient, dismissive, complained that as his hands were unsightly, and looked dirty, he hid them from view when meeting people. He was not amused, or interested, when I made a comment about masturbation, as a boy perhaps, when he was evacuated? Nothing came of this sort of enquiry, except hostility and more tension. The interviews were unpleasant. There was also coolness at present with his mother, who had come from the seaside town to see her other children, but had so far not been in touch with him. He had been too ashamed to write to her after the incident on the beach.

At this moment of impasse, a call came from his wife, troubled once more with cancerphobia, but quickly reassured. She was encouraged by the improvement in her husband's health, he was apparently bearable again. She had long since forgiven him for his infidelity and hoped the problem would now resolve.

At our next session he sat, silent and embarrassed. He complained only of headache, and proposed that as there was so little for us to say, we should stop now. I was hurt, I enjoyed his company, felt his hopelessness and was keen to find out what was the matter with him. I liked him. Was it the handsome features or the challenge of the responsibility I had assumed? Or his wife's attractive eyes shining with confidence in my ability to help them?

He broke my ruminant silence with the announcement that he was worried whether he was doing his work properly (apparently we had that in common). He gazed out of the window and said that as a teenager he had worried a good deal about his parents dying. He spoke of his younger son, his cockiness being out of hand. I mentioned the eczema of the hand again, tactfully, in connection with masturbation. It was no good. He could not accept these theories, he was not interested in these ideas which I for some reason was. And yet, he was still alive, he was back at work, he was back with his wife. But he was pessimistic. "Nothing could be done" by these meetings. We parted amicably, mutually puzzled and I heard no more from him for two years, except via his wife, who continued to call at intervals and say things were not too bad.

Two years later, he asked for another appointment. His job as a production manager was going well but after three years his position became insecure. The firm was being sued about a piece of faulty equipment, the directors were questioning him, he was anxious, unable to work properly. I listened to him, and returned to the timeless themes about responsibility, guilt, the years of separation, the death of his father and its effect on his inner life, his imagination, his feelings.

"I dismiss your ideas," he said calmly. He resigned his job, and was out of work for a while, troubled by eczema.

He is still alive twenty years later, and working, and they have their own flat. The marriage is intact, and his health is good. His wife later developed eczema too, and a duodenal ulcer. Later still two benign lumps were removed from her breasts.

Her mother continued to live with her husband, but mourned her dead lover, buried in the cemetery across the road, near her own father.

"He was a man. He is always in my thoughts. I visit his grave quietly on my own, saying nothing to my husband." she told her daughter.

Most puzzling of all, both the Rogers' sons in this period of time, broke their legs in accidents. The older boy's was complicated and needed pinning. He limped for years, one leg shorter than the other.

7   Brother-in-law

Mrs Lake was pensive, petite and demure. Her husband was tall and burly, a fair haired, pink cheeked coach driver who presided over his family with quiet good humour. Over twenty years, Mrs Lake had given birth to three sons and two daughters. I joined the practice in my twenties, and was the same age as her eldest son: she addressed me as "dear". The family lived in a secluded curved tree-lined street of council houses, near the park: they were built between the wars with generous gardens front and back, and the tenants made good use of them for vegetables, flowers and children's play.

Of Mr and Mrs Lake's children, it was the first and last who worried them most. When the eldest son, Henry, married Sheila, the divorced eldest daughter of the Sumner family, round the corner, the Lakes were not happy. The Sumner's had a reputation for wildness: according to Mrs Lake, it was notorious that Mrs Sumner's children included one fathered while her husband was away at the war — certainly her Fred didn't look like his brothers — and one that was her grandchild.

Mrs Lake's youngest, Brian, always retained his status as the baby of the family: even after his marriage he never looked anything but immature, incomplete, and distracted. His left eye squinted inward, the other looked guardedly out through his spectacles. A crisis overtook Brian, when after the death of the parents, Henry's shadow fell over his marriage.

I had worked in the practice for over ten years, when Mrs Lake came to the surgery with a cancer in her breast, and had a radical mastectomy. Outwardly calm and smiling, she was never reconciled to this hateful insult, which put an end, permanently, to her peace of mind, and to the pleasure she could take in the beauty of her body. Thereafter she was wracked with conflicting anxieties. An undetected return of the adversary could be fatal, and she needed careful supervision. But she felt profound revulsion against being examined and avoided it, until the need for reassurance overwhelmed her. Even then, when she came to it, in the process of undressing and reluctant exposure of the scar, her animosity spilled over onto the doctor, who was made to feel he was an intruder, and violator.

Misfortune continued. Mr Lake, the stout and hearty head of the family, died suddenly from a heart attack within the year, and an affectionate domestic routine ended.

It was about two years after this that Henry Lake, the eldest son, came to the surgery, in deep matrimonial trouble. When he married Sheila Sumner he had thought this childhood sweetheart from round the corner was to be his, after all. He thought he had lost her, or he gave up the idea, when she had someone's baby at the age of sixteen. The infant was, from the very start, brought up by her mother, Mrs Sumner, for Sheila had the family wildness, and was not ready for motherhood yet. She married a soldier next, but that was soon over.

After her divorce, when Henry married her, they were both only twenty one.

When I first met them, they had three children, and I delivered two more, in a poky flat, at the extremity of the practice area, where the land slopes down to the railway junction and the Grand Union canal: down there at that time it was all mean streets and dismal terraces of dilapidated brick, subdivided and sub-tenanted: the clearance of the sites for tower blocks was some years ahead.

The delivery of a baby at night, in dim light, cramped space, on a mattress that sagged, with children peeking round the door, was an obstetric experience which however apprehensive one might be at the time, in retrospect quickly acquired a romantic glow.

The midwife in attendance needed the doctor most often for the repair of a tear, as they were not allowed to perform this minor operation. The opportunities to practice this delicate piece of sewing were infrequent, so that although it was theoretically straight forward, its association to Victorian kitchen table surgery could be uncomfortable. When it was done, and the midwife had tidied up the blood stained linen, the mother given her infant to hold, and the family admitted, the sense of camaraderie was one of the most pleasurable emotional events of the year. The follow up visits confirmed the mutal satisfaction, and were the first steps in the development of a friendship that could endure through another generation.

Sheila, named after her mother, was like a firefly, quick, glittering, small and light. She turned heads, she was pert and tough, with a dangerous gypsy unruliness about her. Henry, named after his father, when in good humour had an easy grin on his sharp red face, with jet black hair combed back and stuck down. He had the gift of the gab, and at night drank more than he could take. By day he was sober, regular in his job on the shop floor, and though generally he appeared agreeably zestful, when he spoke, undertones of sarcasm and paranoia, chilled the atmosphere.

He was the last patient, one evening, it was nearly seven o'clock. He didn't say what was on his mind, probably didn't think I would want to listen, but complained of feeling tense and worried, asked for something to calm his nerves. But for the name on the record card in front of me, I would have overlooked the fact that this haggard, thin lipped, tense man was the son of shy Mrs Lake. There was no family resemblance to his burly genial father.

He came out with it finally: he was being poisoned at work. The story was unclear, I thought at first he meant by an industrial hazard, but he meant deliberate poisoning by some one. This was ominous, perhaps the start of a paranoid breakdown, and I agreed to prescribe a sedative. Later I discovered that this was the first episode in a bizarre series of events that would be the finish of his marriage.

Ten days later, Sheila spoke to me, when she brought in one of their younger children with bronchitis. She told me that some time ago, Henry had come home drunk, and there was a fight, in which their eldest son, a fourteen year old, came to her aid. Henry had accused her, totally unjustly, of going out with another man, insisted that the last baby was not his, that it was a different colour, darker than the others, proof that its father was West Indian. Sheila's gypsy eyes glinted in derision at the idea.

Henry, now off work with depression, told me his version when I asked him what was going on. He confessed he was tormented by the idea of his wife's infidelity, and that the older children were conspiring with her to get him out of the house.

He said that he had put his head in the gas oven, a few months ago, but had changed his mind and decided to take them on and fight. There had been a scene when they had jeered at him, until he went berserk, and he went for the eldest boy with a metal bar. He landed in prison for a month for assault, and it was his own flesh and blood, his wife and children that did it to him.

He knew they had the whip-hand, that they all enjoyed his humiliation, and after another skirmish, when his sons over-powered him, and beat him up with a poker, he moved out. He was determined to go to prison again, rather than pay main-tenance for the child, and would prove that the youngest child was not his, though, as he said, he loved the baby. Meanwhile he was unable to sleep or eat, had lost two stones in weight and spent his time brooding.

As their children grew up, I took an interest in the com-plexion of the youngest, but was never convinced that it was other than pink. Sheila was content to be rid of Henry, who had returned to live with his mother, in her secluded house in the quiet crescent, where his hectic red and black complexion, and morbid character contrasted with the genteel domesticity of his family.

*

Sheila's mother Mrs Sumner, had also been at the surgery worried about pain and stiffness in her fingers. Twelve months before, her husband's stroke had deprived him of speech and the use of his left side, and his wife of much needed support. Mrs Sumner, self contained and plebeian, a neat figure, with a flat London voice, betrayed no sign of the anomalous way of life of which Mrs Lake disapproved. As soon as her children were old enough she had taken a job in a factory canteen, and until these first signs of rheumatoid arthritis, I had seen little of her. She came from a local family who lived in Cross Lane, a secluded strip of sooty street, sealed off at one end by a railway embankment, a neighbourhood of long established residents, where Mrs Sumner's mother, Sheila's grandmother, still lived.

It was bad luck for Mrs Sumner, that in the maisonette beneath her was a demonstration of what severe rheumatoid arthritis was like. An elderly lady, was confined to bed there, knees flexed on her chest, fingers shooting out in all directions, elbows, shoulders, spine, hips, knees all seized up, while her euphoric grin implied merciful mindlessness. She was cared for by her two ambulance driver sons, the district nurse who called every day for years, and compassionate neighbours. She started her disease long before steriods were available, and everything from aspirin to gold injections had failed to halt the mysterious inflammation which finally trussed her up.

Mrs Sumner, when she first showed me her swollen wrists and wasted finger muscles, had said,

"I couldn't bear to end up like that poor woman."

But, soon her knees and hips became inflamed, and within a year the disease was out of control, and she was admitted to hospital. I visited her there once or twice and then once again when her husband suffered another cerebral haemorrhage and died in her absence. Should she leave her hospital bed to attend his funeral? I assumed that with a little assurance she would insist on doing so, but she hesitated, preoccupied with her own sickness. She did go, and returned from the graveside to her hospital bed.

During the next few months at home, a crisis blew up with Alan, her youngest son. He had been a weedy little fellow of six, when I first came to the practice, and he was often brought along by his mother with the coughs and colds and frequent minor injuries. In adolescence he was soon in trouble with the police for petty theft, and his mother showed in her eyes the puzzlement and pain that parents of delinquent children endure. Soon he was injecting himself intravenously with heroin, a registered addict, who spent his time in and out of detention centres and prison.

At the time of Mrs Sumner's admission to hospital, Alan had disappeared from home, and I discussed with her from time to time the possible psychosomatic origin of her rheumatoid arthritis. I spoke of the link between mental and physical pain, and she listened with interest and was grateful for the time we spent together discussing Alan and the possibility of a connection with her illness, since there was no other explanation available.

Her mental state was of unremitting rumination about this unfair and totally incomprehensible affliction, with its end result always tangibly before her in the flat below.

When Alan turned up, his mother was back home, and his father buried. He gave me a sketchy account of his travels, in his twitchy sardonic way, a slight round shouldered young man of about twenty, the smallest of his brothers. He told me he had been to Norway on a fishing trip with some friends, but I always felt he improvised his story as he went along.

He came to ask about his mother, curious in a nebulous way, about the change he observed: she was so thin, and pre-occupied with her disease, at night she wore splints to protect her elbows and wrists from deformity, steroids and gold injections had not arrested the inflammation in her knee and hip joints. Alan was soon in prison again for stealing lead from the roofs of half derelict houses awaiting demolition.

Redevelopment was under way, ill-conceived plans to demolish the Victorian terraces and their gardens and replace them with poor quality flats and tower blocks. Very elderly people after many months of anxiety — no-one could tell them for sure about their future — were forced out of homes and gardens, where they had lived fifty or sixty years. Many failed to survive the shock, and like rabbits flushed out at harvest time went down, not to the farmer's gun, but to the planners' pencil. Twenty years later the planners acknowledged that it was all a mistake, and that refurbishment of the old houses would have been more intelligent. This was a disturbance of the neighbour-hood which went on for about fifteen years. Those with the energy and means cleared out to new towns or neighbouring boroughs to the north. The indigent found themselves isolated in concrete towers, with unreliable and smelly lifts. The elderly infirm were placed in old age homes and geriatric wards.

But the terraces and little streets near the park were untouched, and my visits there to Mrs Sumner and the others continued. Alan, briefly out of prison, arranged for his immediate return there with a childishly transparent cheque forgery. He was sentenced to six years, although was only to serve three. From his cell at Wormwood Scrubs, and later Parkhurst, he corresponded with his mother. She managed a visit, occasionally, and once returned more than usually perplexed. He had asked for a book with a mysterious title. She had no idea what it was or how to obtain any book, and wondered if I could help. It was called — and she searched her handbag for a scrap of paper, and passed it to me — "CAPITAL by Karl Marx." He had also given her a painting by a fellow prisoner, a murderer.

She was appalled by the company he kept, and again I wondered about a connection between her illness and her mental pain. I obtained the book for her, curious to know what he would make of it, but heard no more on the subject. Nor did I hear much from Mrs Sumner about the recent divorce of her daughter from Henry Lake. No doubt she was in pain also, from Sheila, whose wildness had cost her the raising of a grandson.

Her favourite child and chief consolation was Jimmy, a cheerful carpenter, who gave her no trouble, and whose marriage to a motherly handsome girl, worked well. Jimmy's habit of referring to his mother as "the old lady," when he called at the surgery for reassurance about his own hypochondriacal aches, sounded a cheerful note of responsibility and affection.

*

One evening, I was summoned to the nearby home of Mrs Lake. Her eldest son-in-law had died, at the age of forty two, of a sudden heart attack, in the same way as her husband six years earlier. Mrs Lake wept endlessly, unable to speak, and, to my surprise, more visibly upset than by the loss of her husband. The family seemed satisfied to explain this on the grounds that she had been especially devoted to him. Soon there was a transformation from weeping to wheeziness and coughing, signifying the onset of asthma. I was inclined to think of this as emotional in origin, like Mrs Sumner's arthritis.

When the crisis passed, she still breathed with difficulty, and the response to treatment was poor. I sat at the foot of her couch, and tried to comfort her. Perhaps this death might have revived her pain from earlier ones, her husband's, her parents'? She smiled vacantly at this theorizing, and confessed she was more worried about a return of the cancer.

Medication helped her wheeziness no better than my psychological ideas. Her manner continued polite. I was still "dear," but I learned from the family that she sought other advice. Her youngest son, Brian had suggested consulting his faith healer friend. I had met this young man, an ex-male nurse, when he was employed at the local medical equipment shop. I found Brian there once, idling time away with his friend behind the counter. Brian's ambition was to write a hit pop song and I had assumed that his friend was part of that scene.

Brian had complained to me in adolescence of trance-like episodes. He appreciated the chance to talk and a few years later, courting, but depressed, he came again. He spoke of headache, depression, fatigue, chest pains, but finally found the courage to say that he was confused by the fact that his girl refused intercourse:

> "Of course I respect her for it in a way. She's Catholic and says it's wrong outside marriage, her parents were very strict with her. But I'm worried in case it means she's a lesbian. That's what my friend says she might be, anyway."

As this conversation was a few days after I had sent his mother to the hospital with the lump in her breast, I asked him if he knew about it. He agreed it was on his mind, but didn't think there was any connection with his depression.

He was a diffident youth, who never looked virile, even in maturity. His squint made it appear that his attention was half inward, to the world of pop song writing. He worked for the Water Board but said he really hoped to write a successful song. He didn't carry conviction as an artist, musician, poet or even entertainer, nor show any passion for success: it was a dream world, a refuge from pain and the Water Board. In other respects he was unremarkable: in height, build, colour, he was noticeable only for his capacity for invisibility against the background of the throng of humanity.

Earnest, shy, perplexed, he was alternately attracted and repelled by the persistence with which I held to the opinion that he suffered from anxiety rather than anything else. Once he had a fainting attack after indigestion, and with meagre militancy demanded referral to hospital. He was seen by a neurologist, who confirmed the diagnosis of anxiety.

He did not much enjoy his courtship and brooded continually about his fiancée Ann. She had lost her appetite and two stones in weight, and like him, had been sent by her doctor to hospital for tests. I had not yet met Ann but it sounded like anorexia nervosa. Around the time of the wedding, his anxiety increased. He visited me to say,

92

"I feel tired all the time. I feel I'm like my father before he died. He was like this before his heart attack."

The troubled years of his courtship, ran concurrently with his mother's asthma, but whenever he came to the surgery, I was to understand that he wanted more of the talk.

His fiancée Ann did not register at the surgery for some years, but we had met briefly three months after their marriage when she came on behalf of Brian: she was worried about him, he didn't sleep, he had backache, and three times in three months he had wet the bed. Brian for all his doubts about her, seemed to have chosen a pleasant and attractive girl: well spoken and calm, an assistant librarian, able to express her thoughts – but suggesting a feminine version of her husband's abstracted insubstantial presence.

I agreed to talk with Brian again. He added to the list of his problems, perpetual tiredness. He rose early for work, and sat up late to compose:

"I did get one song recorded," he said in a rush of confidence, "but," he slowed down, embarrassed, "the man I was doing it with shot his wife, and then committed suicide."

He had unusual friends, without a doubt. He came to see me once again after a row with Ann: he wanted to make friends with her, but couldn't say so, and was tempted to run away. He asked for and took a small dose of Valium. Neither of them told me that behind their worry about each other was a difficulty in consummating the marriage. Six years later, when Ann registered with the practice, and I received her records, I learned that she had required surgical dilation, and that their baby born two years after their marriage, was born by forceps.

When the baby was one month old, Ann came to see me again, the second time we had met. I thought Brian fortunate in this fair, tall girl but everything about her spoke of girlishness rather than womanhood, her slight figure, solemn blue eyes, dainty features, snub nose, small mouth. She was very worried about Brian again, he was so tense and miserable. This time I spoke to her at greater length about my previous experience of her husband's anxieties and the way they expressed themselves in physical symptoms.

Thereafter I saw little of them for a few years, although this interval was eventful for the Lake family. One year after her son-in-law's death, the hospital chest physician revised his opinion about the nature of Mrs Lake's asthma, and reported to the family possible X-ray evidence of secondary cancer in the chest. I was embarrassed, I had left myself open to misunderstanding with my psychological enquiries. Yet doubt and confusion persisted, both at the hospital and in the family, and I decided not to abandon my position.

Six months later, the hospital diagnosis reverted to a more hopeful option "chronic obstructive airways disease, of unknown origin". Another six months passed before there was unmistakable evidence of secondary cancer. I became a frequent caller then, shown in and out of the family house by her tearful daughters, their good natured cheerfulness overcome by grief, as they attended at the decline and death of that kind, sadly smiling, demure lady.

Her death left the eldest son, Mrs Sumner's ex son-in-law, the resourceful, straight haired, sharp nosed Henry Lake, in possession of the four bedroomed family council house. As this was not acceptable to the Borough Housing Department, it was agreed that Brian and Ann, and two year old Robin, who lived in a one-roomed flat without a garden, should join Henry and keep the house in the family.

The first intimation of trouble from this arrangement, came on one of those visits from Brian with which I used to be so familiar in his youth. I had received two visits from Ann about Brian, now Brian came to tell me he was worried about Ann: they were having ferocious arguments, she was losing weight again, was depressed, and sleeping all day. I suggested that she come round to see me, but she didn't.

One Thursday evening, Brian rang for a home visit. He was worried about Ann, she had lost weight again, couldn't go to work, spent her day asleep on the settee.

On Thursday there was no evening surgery, and requests for home visits disrupted family and leisure hours more than otherwise. I always wanted to discuss the problem on the phone before agreeing to turn out, in an attempt to distinguish panic from genuine medical emergency.

The decisive factor was always mutual confidence. It was

rarely possible to manage this preliminary questioning success-
fully with patients who had no reason to trust my judgement.
Brian, who knew me well, surprised me with the vehement
dismissal of my questions, and was angry when I persisted. He
wanted a visit, and no questions asked.

I found Ann on the same settee, where two years ago, I had
attended Mrs Lake, her mother-in-law. Brian was there,
restless, anxious, glasses glinting hostility.

Ann was mute. Brian again became irritable with me when
I questioned him. I saw that I was not expected to be useful.
Brian was for having her sent to hospital. Ann demurred,
roused herself to mumble that she had a pain in the stomach,
couldn't stand without falling. Two weeks ago, on the
Underground, she had a similar pain. An ambulance took her
to hospital. She had refused vaginal examination there, and
pelvic examination had been done under anaesthesia. She
was told she probably had inflammation of the fallopian
tube.

After a brief examination, I was still mystified. They
reluctantly told me, as if it was a waste of their time, that Ann
had suffered from a mysterious illness dating from the move to
this house, over two years ago. The main symptoms were
abdominal pains, with diarrhoea, intermittent vomiting, and
vaginal discharge. There had been visits to three hospitals, and
all had said the same: there was no evidence of disease, other
than an irritable colon. Valium gave relief, but she was now
drugged all day, and had stopped work. They were defeated,
depressed, sullen and sour. I persuaded them that many
mystery illlnesses were the result of anxiety, and that she was in
no danger at present.

Ann agreed to come to the surgery for further discussion,
during the following week. When she understood that she was
to speak freely, she did:

"I can't stand the atmosphere in that house — it's like a
shrine to Brian's mother. I can't stand having Henry in the
house either. I shall have to leave. Brian won't give up the
house, and I can't stay. If you're right, and it's just nerves,
Brian says I can't have Robin, he won't let me have
custody."

95

I suggested a combined physical and psychological approach as a way out of the impasse, and her dependence on Valium. I would contact the hospitals she had been attending, and arrange for barium studies, while we continued discussions at weekly intervals. I was disappointed, but not surprised when she didn't take up the second part of my offer. She was sensitive to emotional qualities, but I think she felt I was intrusive: she had no concept of psychosomatic illness, could not understand what I meant, and did not trust me much anyway.

Three weeks later, Brian was on the phone again, late on Thursday afternoon, in a replay of the same drama: an unshakeable demand for an immediate emergency visit for Ann's abdominal pain. Frustration conflicted with my curiosity, but I went. I found them exactly as before, and proposed again that while we awaited the results of the X-rays, panic might be avoided by regular appointments for discussion and support. She did finally appear, once more: pale, ethereal, Pre-Raphaelite, depressed and drooping. She addressed me with a vigour and temper, that belied her appearance:

> "You upset me last time. I feel trapped, if it's just nerves. I told you that means I'll have to leave and Brian won't give me custody of Robin."

She wept a little, into a flimsy feminine handkerchief, before she could continue:

> "I tried to cut my wrists last week, but got frightened, and rang my father. He's got a bad heart, I mustn't do that, if I upset him it might kill him. I can't talk to my mother, she won't hear of Brian and me separating, we're Catholic, and neither of them could stand the shame."

She put her handkerchief away, and recovered some asperity.

> "Anyway, I've talked to them now and they know how I feel. It's the house, we should never have moved there, we were quite all right in our flat, except there was no garden. I have to walk in the shadow of my mother-in-law, in that place. Sometimes I even feel I am her. Brian and Henry regard the place as sacred, their sister's the same. Well, I'm not part of that, and they make me feel an intruder into a holy shrine."

She finished on a note of defiance and strength.

"I'm going back to work, anyway. In fact I've already started two days a week, and they can all get on with it."

This was a demonstration of her powers of communication and will. X-ray's of her stomach and bowel were normal. Acceptance of a depressive cause of her symptoms, now named as "living in the shadow of her mother-in-law" encouraged her to return to work at the library after weeks of drugged anxiety. She had been interviewed by the hospital psychiatrist after the wrist cutting episode, and had turned down the offer of a day centre. She did not see herself as a psychiatric patient or even as it turned out, a patient at all. Once again, she broke off contact with me.

Five months later, I was more astonished than irritated when Brian rang one late Thursday afternoon again, in an identical panic. Ann had taken some Valium, and gone to sleep on the couch in the sitting room, awakened, stood up, collapsed, and knocked her head on the fireplace. He had called an ambulance, they had just returned from Casualty. He wanted a visit, immediately, unambiguously. It was unreasonable, but I swallowed my irritation. This unfathomable medical mystery intrigued me, and I went.

The scene was as before: Ann collapsed and mute on the settee, confused hatred flashed from Brian. The reassurance from the hospital doctor had lasted about sixty minutes and then worn off. I explained that they were scared of something which required sustained investigation and discussion, that discontinuity resulted in impasse and panic. I was disconcerted to be told that she had not stopped attending the surgery, she was now under the care of my partner.

She agreed to attend again for discussions. An uncle with schizophrenia, resident in a mental hsopital had died. Terrified, and distrustful of me, she had asked my partner for more Valium. He called in the psychiatrist, who diagnosed depression and offered her the day hospital again. She refused again. Impasse. She reverted to apathy at home, on Valium.

Had she given any more thought to the "the holy shrine"? She half smiled, that seemed fanciful now, she said the problem with the house was really the presence there of Henry, her brother-in-law. She had noticed that her health had improved during a fortnight away from home in Majorca.

A distinct physical agitation went through me, the sensation I supposed called "making the flesh creep". Henry Lake's chill, paranoid personality, the events of ten years ago, his violence in the marriage to Sheila Sumner, came back to me, as revelation:

> " . . . of course . . . . Henry! I had overlooked the connection . . . he lives with them . . . in the same house as this refined young woman, a model of graceful motherhood . . . daily exposed to the barbarian . . . Big Brother to her baffled little brother of a husband . . . "

She described her home under the saturnine rule of Henry. Back from work before Brian, he expected his dinner ready. She did his washing, with that of her own family, and kept his bedroom clean. He frequently got drunk, borrowed money from her and lost it at the betting shop. He teased her, mocked her ill health and timidity. Worst of all was the way he acted towards Robin, as if he knew how to be a better father than Brian. In fact he just confused Robin with over-indulgence one minute, and ill-humour the next. Brian stood by, an intimidated witness to the avuncular ineptitude of his older brother. He was seventeen years younger, and his boyish, dozy personality was no match for a brother of paranoid disposition almost old enough to be his father.

This situation was unalterable, Ann claimed. Henry would never move from the 'holy shrine' into a one bedroomed flat, and leave them alone. If they moved out, Henry would not be allowed to stay by the Housing Department, and the house would be lost to the family. She did show more interest when I pointed out to her, that the question of intrusion was reversed. It was Henry who was an intruder in the "holy shrine" of her married life. She responded at once with the information that young Robin was another problem. He refused to sleep anywhere but in their bedroom, and now that he was nearly five, it had become embarrassing and inconvenient. Robin was a very quiet child who hung behind his mother's skirts when they came together, and he and his mother had a distinctly adhesive relationship. He was another intruder with whom she was contending.

She worried that if she did move out she might be no better off, but was clear that her illness started when they moved in with Henry.

She kept all these thoughts to herself, unable to talk to her husband about it, nor did she much like the trouble I caused her, although she gradually became more thoughtful about her masochistic submissiveness. I left the matter open, asked her to consider it, and perhaps discuss it with the others.

Then an opportunity arose for me to talk to Henry. He collapsed a lung, and was admitted to hospital. When he recovered and came to see me for a certificate, I mentioned his sister-in-law's ill health, in the most general terms. I told him about my theory that his sister-in-law's illness had come about because of the house and its association with the death of his mother, and, I added, that she was missing some of the privacy that married life required. I was of course careful to avoid any personal remarks, but he naturally protested that he was much more of a help to the domestic routine than a hindrance, and could not see that his presence in the house could in any way affect the situation. He was incredulous that he could possibly be in the way, thought that they all got on very well together, but to my relief, agreed that a family discussion was necessary.

When I saw Ann again she looked brighter. There had been some talk at home with Henry, who was now more careful: she noticed he no longer teased her about her Irish parents. She continued to take the Valium, and often vomited a little in the morning, but she told me with some satisfaction that when Henry criticized their upbringing of Robin, she replied that he had seven kids of his own, with whom he had not been too successful!

Now, one by one, other members of the family were drawn in. Henry's sister came to remonstrate that Ann was not being nice to Henry. Ann replied that it was not *she* who had to iron his shirts and clean up his room. Brian didn't have the courage to defend his wife; she hesitated to leave but was worried that her psychiatric history would count against her gaining custody of Robin.

Her mother and father, whom I did not know, came to talk to me, and were astonished at the idea that Henry was the problem. Her mother insisted that it was all due to too many tablets. I talked to them, and they went away, shaking their heads, but promised to help if they could.

When I saw Ann two weeks later, she didn't know her parents had been. She had consulted a faith healer, the one who had helped her mother-in-law. Did I believe in that? No? Neither did her priest who said it was against her religion: Brian had suggested it. She said she had decided to stay with a friend for a week, so that Brian could experience life with Henry by himself.

When she returned, Brian was ready to quit the house. Three weeks later she came to say that she now took fewer tablets, and felt much better. There had been a discussion with Henry, with Brian doing the talking. They had agreed to approach the council together. If they were unable to get a house of their own they would consider emigration to Australia. I suggested that a recommendation from myself and the consultant psychiatrist would help to influence the Housing Department in her favour.

Her parents were puzzled why she hadn't told them that Henry was such a trouble to her, but she herself didn't know until we spoke about it. After each discussion now, she went away feeling hopeful, but confessed to an apprehension that if she did one day have something "really" wrong, I would refuse to come out to her, I would say it was nerves. She agreed ruefully that the reverse of this mistake seemed to be much the most likely in her case.

At Christmas that year, Ann and her family stayed with her parents. Henry joined his sister's family, where he drank too much, and was told that now they understood what Ann had to put up with.

But even after Ann asked me for the medical recommendation for the Housing Department, she hesitated to collect it. Brian came, to demand if it was true that I had said that if they parted, Ann would get custody of the child. He thought it would be judged unreasonable for his wife not to look after his brother. Frightened though he was of Henry, he now realised the danger he was in.

It was May before she saw the psychiatrist, with whom I had already discussed the matter. He told her he agreed with my view of her situation, and that he would supply a letter. She had burst into tears. The case was now before the Community

Physician, to whom I had also spoken, and who undertook to contact the Housing Manager himself.

Ann was now well and working full time, but anxious about the trouble she caused. Did I think she would get depressed again? Henry, who may or may not have been drunk, had made as if to hit her, but instead smashed the top of the fridge. When he made a move towards Robin, she shouted "You touch him and I'll kill you!" There was no longer any question of the marriage breaking up: it was clear that Henry was the problem, and they were united against him.

In July, Ann came in brightly, looking at me with frank and friendly curiosity. The Housing Department had pressed Henry to accept single accommodation, if he refused they would take possession; he doesn't think they are serious about it, but meanwhile is careful not to offend her.

When, on a third visit to the psychiatrist, he questioned her claustrophobia, in the house, she was puzzled. I suggested that he must wonder why she tolerated the situation in the first place. We discussed the delayed consummation of her marriage. She told me that it stuck in her mind as a teenager that a friend was investigated for infertility by having instruments put in down below, and after that she became very scared of internal examinations. She had shared her parents' bedroom up to the age of six, when her younger sister was born. We discussed intrusion into "the holy shrine," from that point of view. She told me that the problem continues in the person of Robin, who refuses to sleep in a room of his own.

She was now beginning to enjoy the struggle to vanquish her opponent. On the day the Housing Department rang she made sure she was out, so that Henry answered the phone. When she returned he looked cross. The next day he went to meet the man from the local council, wearing his best clothes. She heard later that Henry had protested vehemently and claimed that his brother's family were not entitled to re-housing.

Soon after, the family house was surrendered, Henry was satisfactorily re-housed nearby and Ann and Brian and Robin found new accommodation in the suburbs. Ann, no longer "walked in the shadow of the dead", and was freed from her masochistic folie-à-deux with her brother-in-law. Her health and vitality restored, she was ready to contemplate a second pregnancy.

*

Mrs Sumner's story was also nearing its end. She became short of breath and was admitted to hospital in heart failure. She made a slow half recovery, with her weight down to a five and a half stone. When I visited her she told me there had been a fight at home between Alan and Jimmy. Alan had turned up there a few weeks ago with his gypsy-like Irish wife pregnant and nearly at term.

The new baby immediately became a fixture on my visiting list because of his parents' ineptitude. Mrs Sumner senior, was, like the baby, a helpless victim of Alan's incapacity for thoughtfulness. Jimmy, who lived a mile away with his family, kept an incredulous eye on the situation. An argument between the two sons spilled out of the house onto the pavement. Alan picked up a china ornament and threw it through the windscreen of Jimmy's car.

Alan and his family moved out. Mrs Sumner missed the baby, but was relieved.

Then she heard that Alan had rung Jimmy to say that he was back in London but on his own, they had "taken the baby away from him." Said Mrs Sumner, lying in the hospital bed,

"She's kicked him out. It's such a shame. Alan told me he was so happy, that he'd got everything he wanted with his little family. But, there's something wrong with him. Jimmy on the other hand, there's no evil in him."

She looked extremely fragile, with hair cut short, in her make-up and nylon dressing gown. Her limbs were thin as a child's, from wasting of the muscles. She was discharged to be looked after by Jimmy and his wife in their home, and there she died about a year later.

Conrad addressed me with characteristic politeness. He had my full attention, compatible with my awareness that I wanted to like him, but did not find it easy.

His attractive youthfulness and fresh complexion, suggested a healthy mind in a healthy body. The music of his charming slight accent, the pleasing oval of his face, emphasised by baldness, above all that he was the son, the only child, of Mr and Mrs Dabrowska, all these taken together, prepared me to warm to him. But my anticipation was snagged often enough by an indifference in his response. This I put down to his uneasiness with a doctor old enough to be, not his father, but a much older brother.

Not that I saw much of him, sometimes only once a year. Conrad was deputed by his parents, every Christmas Eve to visit the surgery. He would sit patiently in the waiting room, and then when his turn came, enter with a broad grin, gratified by my relief that he had come on a mission of good cheer, rather than professionally. He would then, with some formality and much earnest courtesy, present a bottle of Polish cherry brandy. When he left, bearing my compliments to his mother and father, it was with two or three slight bows, and a degree of awkward uncertainty about the possible discourtesy in turning his back on me to get out of the door.

Now, his politeness was in conflict with unmistakable antagonism that sparked from his handsome blue eyes. His shining scalp gleamed defiance. He hesitated, then plunged:

"You see, sir, it was all right up to last year. Now I have met this girl I would like to marry, but it is impossible if I am like this. I will tell you what I think, although of course, sir, I am not a doctor. I was abstinent in sexual matters up to two years ago, but after that not so much, and I am wondering if it is possible I could have damaged myself in some way? You will know better than me."

He awaited an answer. I irritated him by my hesitation, my uncertainty as to what exactly he was talking about, by my not knowing immediately what he meant. He had exerted himself to get this far, and was not prepared, or able, to go into the minutae: it was embarrassing enough already. The scalp gleamed a warning that the time I was alloted to guess the answer was running out.

I told him I thought of it as a psychological problem, not related to infection, or damage from sex, and that I would find it helpful if he could talk to me more about it. It was his turn not to understand what I was talking about.

I suggested we might talk about his life situation in general, but he was not with me, and I found that it was becoming increasing difficult for me to explain. I wanted to tell him that there was a theory, which I found useful, that sexual difficulties were part of a more general problem between people wanting to relate to one another, and that the method of finding out more about it was through the medium of discussion, in the hope that with patience and thought, something might come up that would help.

I think his difficulty was with the concept of "psychological". He was rising rapidly in his work through the lower managerial ranks in a factory where the weak were left behind, and the successful achieved rapid material rewards. Although I knew his parents, and had come to like and admire them, communication with them was also difficult. His father's English was absurdly bad, considering how long he had been exposed to it. His mother's was good, she was a communicator, a talker and letter writer, and proud, rejecting any attempt, however well intentioned, to breach the privacy of her domestic life.

Even later, when she and her husband were grievously upset by Conrad's misadventures, and our friendship was secure, it was almost impossible for her to take me into her confidence about it. Perhaps her letters to Poland to her sister, were the secret of her apparent self containment in emotional matters.

Conrad struggling with bafflement and suspicion, tried out my suggested method,

"My parents are very peculiar about such matters, sir. It was impossible for me as a child to talk with them about sex. Even now, they don't make it easy for me to bring a girl home. If I do they are always criticizing her as not being good enough for me, or else she is too plump, or too short." He snorted derisively, "Sir, it is quite ridiculous, they are very possessive of me. They are childish, they think if I get married, I will no longer take care of them."

He was an eloquent accuser of his parents. This pained me, considering that I thought Mrs Dabrowska had nobility of character, a Polish Mother Courage, and that I liked his father's upright bearing, ironic good humour, and invincible constitution, as well as his eccentric pronunciation, and antiquated continental courtesy.

Conrad's deference was a pastiche of his father's puntilio in the matter of greeting and departing. His manner of leaving the consulting room, must have been correct etiquette in the time of Stanislaw II: up from the chair, to attention, click of the heels, brisk military bow, and without hesitation out, backwards. If his mother brought the Revolutionary Study to mind, with his father it was Pan Taduska.

Conrad was able to overcome his distaste for my method of enquiry, sufficiently to accept that his problem required more time for exposition and definition. He agreed to come back at the end of the evening surgery.

Our talks were just round the corner from his parents' house, in the old surgery, since demolished. The consulting room, once a Victorian doctor's drawing room, was unexpectedly spacious for a district of crowded terraces and narrow streets. Now it was stripped of its original oak veneer pannelling, and the walls painted utilitarian grey, decorated with a couple of reproduction still lifes: Cezanne oranges, a Matisse sideboard with jug.

The desk stood before a grey marble fireplace, whose fire was no longer set, heat came from an electric bar radiator when required. On the mantel were a few homely trophies, gifts from patients: a painted wooden pen stand from the West Indies, a pottery cockerel from Portugal, a black painted elephant from Ceylon, and a little hand carved wooden box from Poland, a present from Conrad's mother.

The furniture was modest: a couch, a cabinet of drugs and

dressings, a little table with sterilizer and instruments, the desk with sphygnomanometer and telephone, innumerable pens and papers, the chair at the right hand side for the patient and on the left for an escort, the little buzzer tacked to the left hand desk panel to call the next patient. The impression was somewhat dowdy, even a little depressed, consonant with the neighbourhood.

Conrad was touchy, his jaw pointed at me, his naked scalp glistened. He was sceptical of men in office, of status conferred by a chair behind a desk. He had pulled back his chair from its place at the right of the desk, to a strategic distance from which he scrutinised me, looking for evidence to confirm his suspicion that I was out of my depth. His complexion, smooth and brown, his bright blue eyes, the gleaming scalp, required of me an answer. Was I or was I not familiar with the territory in which he had lost his way? As a boy during the Second World War he had travelled as a refugee with his mother from Siberia to India. He had learned not to waste time with irrelevant people, irrelevant to survival. A few words and a glance were enough to tell whether to move on, try someone else, somewhere else. He had learned to forage, to conserve energy, not to expect anything to come from wasting time, negotiating with the obtuse.

I was cautious, I wanted to catch his interest and prolong the discussion. He considered impotence to be like pneumonia: as if to say 'if you have something useful to tell me, out with it; if not, if you're out of your depth, admit it, and have done'. He was an engineer, not street wise, but wordly wise, and world war wise. The clean lines of his temples, the glossy scalp, the bright eyes, glinted with intelligence: I saw him in imagination, at ten years old, on the epic journey from Russia to India, suddenly break way from his mother's side to reconnoitre. After fifteen years in England, his accent was slight, an unfamiliar, but pleasing rhythm. His foreign courtliness, holding out under strain, was his father's: the obstinacy, his mother's.

Her hypochondria, like her osteoarthritis, was at an early stage when we first met: in those days she walked to the surgery and put up with the waiting room. Once seated by the desk, she gave detailed, repetitive accounts of the discomfort in her joints, and didn't conceal her scepticism about pain relieving tablets.

She was in fact in the early stages of osteoarthritis, but it was the perseverance of her lament, the tenacity with which she held to her theme, and her refusal of assent to hopefulness, that penetrated my hide, stirred up irritability and criticism. Obstinacy and suspicion had equipped her for survival in the maelstrom.

Fine sad blue-grey eyes scrutinised me, as did Conrad's at a later date, for signs of insincerity; she sat in the bentwood chair by the desk, upright, a queenly presence, unpacifiable in connection with her demand for attention to the pain in her fingers, in her hips, in her knees, in her neck: pains as yet giving little away in visible, palpable evidence of swelling, inflammation or deformity, elusive diagnostically.

Her abundant white hair, once flaxen, she gathered into a chignon: on home visits, in the years ahead, I saw it free and waist length: she trailed her clouds of glory still. But now, at the time of our early acquaintance, it was unclear to me what this phenomenon, Mrs Dabrowska, had in store for me. Her beauty was clear, the clean lines of her bone structure ensured that ageing was unable to spoil her appeal to the eye, rather made her attractiveness more complex, maternal.

But hypochondriacal complaining is wearying to the ear, however much the eye is gratified by appearance. Something exhausts compassion in the listener, the note of self pity, the egocentricity that lies so cunningly hidden within. The doctor is a practical man, he wants to make contact with something solid, some reality either of mind or body. The complaint in hypochondria is a Proteus, it slips and slides from the grasp.

Her Polish inflection tripped and faltered as she struggled to make English sense from Polish syntax. I listened, restless and wondering, to her reiterated descriptions of the pain, and her objections to every kind of tablet, her suspicion that I was not interested, not attentive, that I was an *apparatchik*, a medical official, making a living out of useless if not poisonous pills.

I hung on, maybe admiring her looks, more than listening to all the ins and outs of her complaints. But she needed a listener, not an admirer. She was in pain, and there was evidence of an early stage of that osteoarthritis of the fingers and knee and hip joints that some complain of more than others. But her pain was not all arthritis, and never was. The more I listened, the more I fell under her spell. I became curious about her, attracted to

107

her personality, her way of expressing herself, as well as the splendour of her profile. As I allowed myself to be borne along, I realised that I was no longer feeling persecuted by her complaints.

She too, had altered, the lines about her mouth were softer, she was looking out at me, as well as inward at her bad luck. She had begun to notice me, as I had noticed her. Her voice became more musical, she ceased to complain, became confidential, friendly, appreciative. She was indeed a handsome matriarchal figure, who had encountered communists, Nazis, and others, and come through, though not unscathed. Before any outward sign of severe arthritis, she feared immobility: survival had depended on being able to move on, to get away. She walked without a stick then; in the years ahead, this trans-continental voyager was beaten by the staircase, narrow and steep, that spiralled to her upstairs living quarters. Imprisonment there became inevitable,as her hip joints gradually crumbled. When she could no longer come to me, I visited her regularly. I was under her spell.

The Dabrowska's house was slotted between higher and wider ones, faced, not like the others, with brick, but with white cement. A shop once, it now looked like a child's drawing, with windows in flat iron frames, and a green painted front door. Its idiosyncrasy symbolised displaced Poles lodged amongst the English.

It was a friendly street, on a homely scale, narrow, so that heavy traffic avoided it. Terraces of brick villas, with decent sized rooms, accessible front doors, and neighbours who stopped to talk; a hundred years old, the two lines of fifty villas looked at each other across twelve yards of cobblestones, each protected by a minute area of fenced forecourt in front of the parlour window. Indoor toilets and bathrooms were only now being added by many of the owners, while tenants with fixed rent, struggled with reluctant landlords in the hope of — unprofitable — improvements.

My weekly talks with Conrad about his impotence, did not go smoothly. I was not convinced by his theory that his mother wanted to stop him from marrying. I perceived her as the epitome of grandmotherliness. Perhaps he really was bringing home "unsuitable" girls? Inevitably he began to idenfity me with his parents, with whom he was unable to "talk about sex". But he at least accepted that the problem was in the mind, and thought it was logical that I should refer him to an appropriate clinic for psychotherapy. He was not willing to continue the discussions with me, and I agreed to refer him.

For a year or two I saw very little of him although I understood from his mother's vague hints that certain developments had upset her. The treatment at the clinic must have enabled Conrad to marry the girl, but he immediately discovered, according to his mother, that he had been tricked. His Polish wife had merely wanted to acquire British nationality, and had deserted him almost at once.

With the advance of her arthritis, and her age, Mrs Dabrowska gradually established a sanctuary for herself in her front bedroom. From there, her refuge, she conducted her affairs with the outer world, coming out only when the ambulance called to take her to the hospital for physiotherapy. In the summer, she sat at the window in her peignoir, hair coiled, to observe the street life below, as village elders do the world over: neighbours hurrying here and there, young men working on cars, children at noisy play, dogs, cats, sparrows, shadows of the roof tops in sunshine. Her own creamy cat Cashka, was never far from her.

She slept in a single wooden frame bed in the corner near the window. Her husband slept in his own room off the landing. On her simple dressing table, amongst the scattered sewing materials, combs and creams and tablets, were pamphlets and paperbacks in Polish. On top of a small pinewood wardrobe, two canvas suit cases, travel stained, had come to rest. An armchair by the window marked her observation post. Convenient to hand on a low table by the bed, beside more bottles of paracetamol and indomethacin, and the tube of Algipan embrocation, were her pocket Polish-English dictionary, notepaper and pens: correspondence with Poland and arthritis in her fingers were her antagonistic, twin pre-occupations. Above the white painted mantelpiece with its assortment of little ornaments: a poster in Polish, donated by Conrad, who was in possession of all the downstairs rooms.

These I never entered, and the doors were never left ajar. Conrad was never at home on my visits, or ever ill, and he worked long hours.

In her boudoir, ancient wallpaper matched the faded green of a worn Indian carpet and of her bedspread. Her calendar, with seascape, fastened by a drawing pin to the wall by her bed, showed certain some days in red, but the significance of these dates belonged to a culture I did not know. One other room completed the living quarters upstairs, a small kitchen at the back overlooking a square of overgrown garden. Occasionally I would find Mrs Dabrowska seated there at the table, with the debris of a meal. The kitchen was common ground with her husband, who undertook the shopping and the elementary cooking on the battered gas stove, and washed up afterwards at the earthenware sink.

There were no faded photographs of parents or new colour ones of children, as in the living rooms of her neighbours. All seemed to declare her exile, and transposition, grafted into the life of the street, out of line, like her house. Yet, evidently her unusual character, and I think her beauty, attracted the interest of others, beside myself. Her neighbours were conscious of her presence amongst them, were sympathetic to her problems, and worried about her. They saw her as a transcendent version of their own parents or grandparents, who could recall the green fields and country lanes in North London, as she remembered her village in Northern Europe.

My monthly visits lasted only ten minutes, but I enjoyed them, charmed by her comeliness, awed by her history. Her hair that was flaxen, and was now white, was frequently allowed its freedom rather than be coiled into the chignon, and although her oval face with those melancholy blue grey eyes maintained their customary gentle glance and her complexion remained clear, she was irked by her increasing immobility, arthritic hands, grating knee and hip joints. In later years she became careless of her appearance, and it was about that time that I would find her more often sitting in the back kitchen disconsolate amongst the debris. By then she had lost interest in the street at the front and rarely looked out at the little back garden, with its solitary walnut tree and overgrown patch of grass.

My knock on the front door was answered after a short delay, by Mr Dabrowska. His English pronunciation was staccato, opaque and obscure in a stutter of interpolated consonants. He was a lean man at this time, about seventy, with a straight back, grizzled face, darting brown eyes, and a smooth scalp. His greeting was always warm, vocal, but unintelligible. The basis of his greeting and parting ritual was the sharp inclination of the head at attention, and the click of the heels. Consecutive conversation being so difficult, Mr Dabrowska often acted an ironic pantomime, to express his feelings about life.

There was an indoor version, and an outdoor. The former was restricted by the space available, and possibly inhibited by the presence of his wife. There was very little reaction between them, no arguments, no outward show of affection. But when he went into his pantomime routine, she was not amused.

The outdoor version took place outside his front door as he accompanied me to my car: he would set off, erect, and shouldering a phantom rifle, to march a few paces up and down the pavement, oblivious to passers-by:

"In Poland I was Teacher, Headmaster. Chemistry, Science. Then came War. Teacher no more, Soldier I must be. March up and down, salute, learn shoot, Bang, bang, march, always march. No, I tell them. Me teacher, not soldier. But I must be soldier. For ten years, I am soldier. Must march and shoot. Bang, bang!"

A grin and a handshake. The stiff bow. The clicked heels. Then he stood there until I was out of sight. This Brechtian improvisation was an effective piece of sardonic street theatre, which put over his story with admirable brevity. I noticed from my rear view mirror as I drove off that he stood for several seconds gazing after me before turning back into the little house.

I often tried often to draw out from him a less abridged edition of his life story, but without success. He had the greatest difficulty in speaking English, other than part he had learned for his performance. If I persisted, he would have to turn to his wife and ask her in Polish to give me an answer. In this way I did learn more, but from her point of view, which was not the same.

He dressed badly, in old baggy trousers and a collarless shirt. For shopping he put on a dilapidated raincoat and a ruined trilby hat, which gave him the appearance of a tramp. As he dragged along with two shopping bags, women avoided him, and children stared. The neighbours were united in finding Mrs Dabrowska lovable, and her husband bizarre, unapproachable, and unhygienic.

One day in the front room, in a more cheerful, animated mood — she had a letter that day from her younger sister in Cracow — Mrs Dabrowska was willing to tell me more about their story. Her husband stood by, tea cloth in hand, following the narrative, nodding, smiling and exclaiming as the narrative unfolded. Her father had been a forester in the area around Cracow, who liked to carve small wooden boxes and figures in his spare time. Like her mother before her Mrs D. trained as a primary school teacher. When she was 26 she married a schoolmaster from a neighbouring village, and they had one son, Conrad, who was nine when the Red Army, on its way to stop the Germans invading Poland from the West, overran their home.

They were deported to Siberia. In the summer of 1942, General Anders, released from Lubjianka prison, in Moscow, formed his army of Polish prisoners of war and deportees, and set out for the Middle East: Mr. D. was with them. His wife and son followed later with other families, on the long trek to India, via Iran. Transport was slow, conditions hazardous, but they arrived safely and stayed in India until after the war when they were re-united in England.

There was a short stay in temporary camps in the Midlands, and then they were able to buy the little house in London. Hence my romantic view of her as Mother Courage: unbowed victim of human stupidity, invading armies, hypocritical politicians and careless bureaucracy, who embracing her child, defied Russians and Germans, traversed Europe and the Middle East and India on slow trains, survived in tents and transit camps, presided over Conrad's development, and in England organised his education.

Conrad was never to be seen at home, or any trace of him. His mother had only once hinted at a disastrous marriage. But doubt on this version was cast by Conrad himself, when six months after my conversation with his mother, he came to the surgery, very irritable indeed.

He was worried by chest pain, and the possibility of a heart attack, but when I had satisfied him on that issue, his expression darkened, anxiety gave way to fury. He pulled from his wallet a typed letter, a statement signed by the consultant psychiatrist at the clinic to which I had referred him. The last paragraph read:

" . . . . *Treatment was completely successful, so that he was able to perform the sexual act on numerous occasions over the eighteen months from June 19. . . to January 19. . .*

This document, fumed Conrad, had been crucial evidence in his fiancée's decision to marry him. Yet in the end he had been unable to consummate, and she had left. He was simmering with resentment that I had sent him to a clinic, "where they were all homo's".

Whether his version or his mother's was correct, I never found out, but perhaps it was a combination of both. He was as alienated from his parents as ever. There was a new note of contempt in his remarks about his father, whom he claimed was becoming senile. Up to this time I had always thought that of the three, it was Conrad who was most disturbed, and I discounted his remarks about his father as an aspect of his psychological difficulties.

But other evidence pointed in a different direction. I heard later from his mother that Conrad had married again, and this time all was well. Soon after, on a routine visit to their house, the old man took my arm and led me to the back kitchen. He pointed out a small dark damp stain on the ceiling, and with much gesturing and uttering, conveyed that he wanted to demonstrate the method by which his neighbours caused rainwater to be conducted from their roof, to his lower lying one.

I was disconcerted to discover that he had finally accused his neighbours of this absurdity: accosted them on the pavement with some kind of incoherent fuss. They spoke to me about it, said they were sorry for the old lady who was sweet, but that her husband was a pig. I thought this was harsh, but I did not live next door to him, merely continued to enjoy his eccentricity.

There had recently been a moving reunion in the little house. Mrs. D.'s niece from her native village arrived on a visit. This lady, daughter to Mrs D's late sister, had a child of the same name and age as one of mine. Mrs. D had made much of this, photographs had been exchanged and items of interest had been reported in the correspondence with her niece, who brought little gifts for the home nurse's family and for mine. The ambience in the upstairs room when I was introduced was wonderfully emotional. Joy and excitement, sorrow and distress: a unique occasion, this memorable meeting, the first since the family left home twenty years ago, and also the last time they would see each other.

As the nurse and I – privileged to attend at this painfully joyous re-union – communicated our solidarity with the universal values of family life, Mr. D. poured little glasses of Polish vodka, clicked his heels, and smiled the smile that was probably only partially sardonic, and repeated *sotto voce* in his litany, his difficulty in assimilating what fate had decreed for him:

"In Poland I am teacher. No, they say must be soldier, I must march, march. I not soldier, am teacher, science, chemistry, but they say 'March'! So I march!"

Time added heart failure to Mrs D's arthritis. There were gloomy discussions about her future. Conrad had his living to make, Mr. D. was not capable of the effort requried to look after an invalid. He shuffled and pattered about in the little upstairs kitchen, cooked an omelette, heated soup, nothing to stimulate a failing appetite, and was soon tired by the steeply winding little staircase, that trapped his wife upstairs. There were visits to the physiotherapy department and several temporary admissions to the geriatric ward, when the ambulance men threaded her down the narrow stairs, strapped to a chair, and struggled up with her again on her return.

In the ward, I generally found her by her bed, unhappy at the lack of attention she received from the harassed staff. The strains of Chopin's Revolutionary Study seemed further away. On the bedside table where her pen and paper and dictionary lay within reach, amongst the fruit, flowers, and talcum powder, she continued to fight the war between personal human warmth and the organized bureaucracy in which the well meaning nurses were so often trapped. But her hair, now leached of colour, had been cut short, and she was less substantial, as if regular bathing and nursing had removed the sinew and muscle that supported her: less travel stained, but infinitely more vulnerable; hygienic, but unhappy, she wanted to be home.

A year later, it was time for her to move to the long stay geriatric hospital. She seemed alert, but when her possessions went astray, and they often did, she was quick to suspect theft. She lost her spectacles, there was a long delay before they were replaced, and her letter writing was interrupted. Amongst the twenty other women there, some still held out against dementia. She made a friend of one, and on one of my visits introduced us:

"This is my doctor," she said with possessive pride and held my hand while we talked. But she was unsure if the staff would approve, and her glance down the ward, where nurses were working, showed her anxiety that she might infringe an order of the day or incur disapproval for this sign of emotional weakness, for seizing hold of the chance to express affection. That moment quickly passed, no-one seemed to mind, we spoke of the children, and of her husband and Conrad, both of whom visited her frequently. She also had visits from a few Polish friends and from the Home Nurse, over whom she had also cast her spell, during the years of invalidism in that little house.

She became thin, an advantage with arthritis, but definite hints of incipient dementia was obtruding. Much more of her conversation was in a persecutory mode: the nurses were deliberately ill-mannered and rough with her, her possessions were being pilfered. The death of her friend in the ward, left her without energy for new friendships, she became quiet and apathetic. No more letters were written to Poland. I continued to visit her, but at longer intervals. She remembered less and less of her former life, but each time I left she ensured that I would return to her bedside, by murmuring " . . . . don't forget me" as I slipped my hand out of her tight grip.

These were difficult years for Conrad. I never met his second wife with whom he lived downstairs in the little house. The responsibility for his father upstairs affected his health, and he appeared at the surgery with chest pains again, and with indigestion. There was no doubt now that the old man was demented and paranoid. He walked the streets in bedraggled rags, the old hat pulled low over his brow, his gaze in the gutter. His grasp of English had weakened until he let go of it altogether.

His unwashed flesh and bent spine evoked defeated soldiery, a ghostly remnant of a routed army, that looked in the mud and snow for a homeward path. Passers-by saw a crack-brained tramp. The headmaster of pre-war days was much reduced.

His smelly place upstairs and his unsanitary presence were hard for Conrad and his wife to bear. He came round one evening to give me a dossier of his father's antics. This document, neartly written out in blue ink, covered several sides of notepaper and was headed in capital letters:

"A BRIEF MENTAL HISTORY OF MY FATHER."

Its purpose was to present to the authorities the case for his father to be certified insane. I had been reluctant to believe that a mental hospital was the best place for his father and resisted Conrad in this. I did not like the obstinacy and apparent indifference with which he had held to his occupancy of the ground floor of the house, and thus forced his parents to live upstairs and his mother to be trapped up there. Without the obstacle of that impossible staircase she would have enjoyed access to the street, it was as bad as a lock and chain on the front door to her. Yet she would never hear of Conrad being approached to exchange floors. She was frightened of him in some way, she did not want to meddle with him, or ask him to become involved with her problems. She wanted to spare him.

I entertained briefly the idea that it was Conrad who was the psychiatric patient, and recalled his long standing contempt for his father. Now that his mother was in the geriatric ward, was his next move to get his father locked up in a mental hospital, and take the whole house for himself?

Yet "A Brief Mental History of My Father," made out a strong case, if true. It listed such items as: "hostility to neighbouring houses, with accusations that they are damaging the property. Accusations that I steal his clothing, and prolonged intrigues against me when visiting mother in hospital." (Interesting! I had not appreciated when I had seen him shuffling down the road that he was capable of getting there on his own, it was at least six miles away, and difficult to reach across some dangerous main roads.) Then there was "persistent talking and shouting, day and night, about me wishing to have them dead or cheat them." Other items related to a fixed

116

delusion that there was a man in his room, who patted him on the head and back, and an impossibly involved conglomerate of paranoid suspicions about a missing Old Age Pension book, which was in his pocket all the time. In short, it was a damning indictment of his father, rather than a brief mental history, and the end of his liberty was near.

Neighbours whom he had offended put their oar in, social workers appeared, the police picked him up far from home, when he lost the track that had been leading him to his wife's bedside. He had forgotten the name of the hospital as well as how to reach it.

He was removed to spend the remainder of his life in a geriatric mental hospital. I concluded I had been unjust to Conrad who now behaved with exemplary conscientiousness. When we met, we spoke about them.

"Its pathetic, sir. Last week I took my father from the mental hospital to visit my mother. She took him for her father, and he thought she was his mother!"

Old Mrs Dabrowska died first, after nearly six years in the geriatric hospital. Her husband continued to exist, with wisps of thought echoing through his vacant mind, about teaching science, marching and saluting, and about the search for his lost wife and mother . . .

9   Mrs Spriggs' ordeal

One cold night in February, at 2.a.m., Mr Spriggs, a genial youthful figure, who might have been taken for a benign schoolmaster, but was in fact a railwayman in his forties, was killed by a train as he worked on the track in a tunnel between Hendon and Colindale.

The Coroner was critical of the safety precautions taken by London Transport, but Mrs Spriggs blamed the flagman. It was his duty to warn oncoming trains of the presence of workmen. She was convinced that if the facts were as the flagman gave them at the enquiry, he would also have been taken unawares and killed with her husband.

Her husband's death had a catastrophic effect on Mrs. Spriggs. She lost all initiative, refused to eat or walk, or do anything other than smoke, weep, and get drunk. She began to shrivel and shrink, her face screwed up like a squashed lemon, she lost weight, her clothes hung on her: she slept in them on the sofa in the sitting room where the curtains were never drawn back. She wanted to die, threatened that she had a loaded revolver in the house, but wouldn't say where. Her frightened neighbours and relatives insisted that I call a psychiatrist: he offered to admit her into a hospital, but she refused.

Some weeks passed. Obsessed with the accident, she ruminated endlessly on certain mysterious aspects. There were specific safety regulations always strictly enforced. All men involved with work on the line were trained to treat the occupational hazard with the greatest seriousness, and to follow carefully the safety regulations. Her husband, of all men, was careful, cautious and responsible. He was not the type to take any chances.

Her suspicions hardened, and now widened to include another man, not only the flagman, but also Ted, her husband's workmate. She waited for the inquest, losing weight, smoking, weeping, crushed.

The attitude of her friends shifted. The flood of sympathy spent itself. Her response to commiseration was cool. They found her suspicions morbid, her pre-occupation with self destruction frightening, repellent, macabre. A neighbour remembered, and told another psychiatrist, called in by an apprehensive social worker, that Mrs Spriggs had always been too dependent on her husband. Her only relative in London, also a patient of the practice, did what she could to help, but her husband, finding that his wife was ill with worry about her cousin, lost patience with Mrs Spriggs and shouted at her,

"Well, why don't you go and kill yourself, if it's that bad?"

The impasse was broken by the decision that she should go for a holiday to the home of her younger sister at the coast. When she came home, a few weeks later, I received a notification from the health authority that she had changed doctors, accompanied by the usual request for the return of her medical records.

The loss of a patient hurts, even if there has been little satisfaction in the relationship. But Mrs Spriggs and her husband had always been on the most cordial terms with me. I wondered if I had been tactless like her cousin's husband, or whether she was just cutting off because I reminded her of her life with her husband.

It was true that Mrs Spriggs lived some distance away across the North Circular Road. Like so many patients of this old established practice — its doors were first opened nearly a hundred years ago — she had moved away from the immediate area without changing doctors.

The surgery was in a depressed economic and social locality, with crumbling housing and inadequate roads for the ever increasing traffic. Many families, as soon as they were able, moved out to cleaner, fresher, more spacious areas but kept the family tie with the practice. The emotional link held, despite the health authorities regulation which tried to quantify the mileage over which a doctor's responsibility could reasonably expect to stretch.

There was an amusing aspect to these impractical arrangements. They were coldly regarded by any new doctor at the practice, irritated by a request for a visit to a distant part of the borough, when they were on call. But of course, new doctors soon found themselves caught up in the same sort of dilemma as they made their own emotional ties to patients, and in their turn suffered the incomprehension of newcomers ...

120

I didn't forget about Mrs Spriggs and her tragedy, her cousin gave me news of her at intervals. Nothing dramatic was happening, I gathered.

A year later a letter came on lined paper torn from a cheap pad. The hand that wrote it trembled, but the letters were neat and round, correctly sloped slightly to the right,

"*Dear Dr.*

I am writing to ask if you will please take me back on your books.

I really did it on the spur of the moment. I was so ill at the time and I thought the other doctor was nearer, but I have no confidence in him.

I would be grateful if you could do this for me,

Thanking you

Yours sincerely

Mrs F Spriggs

P.S. Could you let me no as soon as possible because I am sorry I ever left you."

I felt relieved and thankful that the link held: in retrospect I wondered about her uncharacteristic spelling mistake. I wrote back at once with my agreement. Then came a second letter: she had a hospital appointment to see the psychiatrist, was refused transport, but was unable to wait for buses because she "came over faint".

She had no telephone: I decided to visit her. She lived in a semi-detached council house, built between the wars, off the North Circular Road. The streets are leafy and secluded. The area was planned and constructed at the time of the Wembley Exhibition of 1926, when the country lane that led to Wembley was widened into a four lane thoroughfare. One eighty year old man told me he remembered the old road being so narrow that as a boy he had squeezed against the hedge to avoid a pony and trap. Room for two or three streets of houses at that time was tucked into land that was reclaimed from London Transport for their employees. It was a parcel of land that remained surprisingly sheltered from the storms of traffic that thundered nearby.

That afternoon, Mrs Spriggs' avenue was peaceful. Some workmen opposite her house had put up scaffolding and were clambering about, whistling as they re-tiled the roof. An arthritic old man in a cloth cap hobbled by and was overtaken by

121

two young women with prams, and shopping bags.

The sound of their footsteps receded. Mrs Spriggs was slow to answer my knock, the bell was not working, her curtains were drawn. It was early March, the sun failed to give any warmth: in the chill of her porch, it occurred to me that I might regret taking her on again. I thought I heard a shuffle inside, but minutes passed before the door slowly opened. She had lost more weight, shrivelled up even more, since I saw her twelve months ago. Her hair was uncombed, her clothes rumpled. She apologized — had been asleep on the sofa — turned and groped her way back to the shadowing smoky sitting room, where she bedded herself down in the armchair. A twenty two inch TV at her elbow, blocked her view to the right. At her left was her settee, her bivouac: messed up bedclothes, litter of papers, greasy plates, cigarette debris, dust everywhere: she was like a shade, the familiar of a haunted place, not of the world of the living, outside the front door.

"I'm glad you've come — I just had a nose bleed."

Her voice was flat, matter of fact, stronger than I expected. She waved one nicotine stained hand at the litter of bloody Kleenex tissues around her feet, and dabbed at her nose with the other.

I sat down opposite and listened to her story. She complained of dizziness and inability to walk, her neighbours no longer called, she would be better off back in hospital. She had been in a psychiatric ward for six weeks and was to have attended at the Day Hospital. Her refusal to use public transport had led to an impasse.

As I sat and listened to her I began to understand that I was called in now because she had long since alienated all sources of sympathy, other than her cousin. She had repented of her initial refusal of psychiatric help, and experienced the protection of the psychiatric department. On balance she preferred her own home. But she had exhausted and exasperated the hospital staff in the end. The passive helplessness that demanded constant support and attendance of all kinds and from all-comers had exhausted the tolerance and sympathy of everyone, doctors, neighbours, relatives, social workers. Her ill-fortune and depression were hard enough to contemplate, but this ego-tistical apathy aroused disgust and animosity. Sulky, wounded, unpleasant to approach: like a parasite, she could batten onto you, burrow into you, lodge herself under your skin or in your mind, until you were ill yourself.

Her mental energy was reserved for deciphering the enigma of the accident that killed her husband, there was none to spare. She showed me the newspaper cutting of the inquest, found it immediately among the litter of papers on the sofa: she was organised to conduct that business, and no other. The newspaper report mentioned the medical evidence, the impact of a train at speed, multiple injuries ... She sat hunched up, pulled at her cigarette and spoke of compensation, then her nose started to bleed again. I tried to plug it with a rolled up tissue, but the blood came from her obsession with her husband's corpse, her identification with it.

I had known her husband well as a patient at the surgery, a pleasant, friendly, slim, good humoured man. I sympathised with her refusal to let him go without a fuss, without enquiry, without compensation, without complaint. They had met after the war. Her family were villagers in Kent. After school, she went as a maid to a house in Bromley. During the war she worked in a munitions factory. It was once strafed by a marauding plane: she had a scar over her right eye still, from a fall when they all ran to the shelter.

After the war, she went back home and lived with her mother until her death. She was thirty-six when her older sister from London introduced her to her future husband. A hysterectomy for fibroids ruled out children. In the three years before the accident she had lost a brother and sister and her father. There was only one younger sister left.

There was no food in the house, she was scared of the nose bleeds, she wanted to go into hospital. I was due to start a holiday the next day, and I arranged her admission before I left. When I returned two weeks later, I found the problem still there. The hospital had not admitted her, just plugged her nose again and sent her back the same night. That weekend she had taken an overdose of her depression tablets, been seen in Casualty, kept in overnight and sent home again. A neighbour called in my partner. He asked the psychiatrist to come again: when he offered admission, she refused.

Impasse: she wanted something, called for help, expected

someone to do something, but what? Not hospital now, apparently. She complained of her neighbour, who would no longer take any responsibility for her, but forbade her to go to her sister, who was ill. A patina of psychotic thought was noticeable: Mrs Spriggs suspected a plot, thought she would take a taxi to the coast to find out the truth. She showed me another newspaper cutting, a report of the London Transport enquiry into the accident, and was sceptical still, convinced there was a cover up, the truth had not yet come out.

She sat sideways on the edge of her cretonne covered armchair, amongst the debris of her domesticity: no stockings, slippers down trodden, slept-in housecoat, hair straggly, face squashed, cigarette end expiring in an ashtray, the packet shoved out of sight under the cushion. She squinted up at me as I stood bewildered before her: there was nowhere to sit for the purpose of conversation. The TV was up against one arm of her chair, at the other she had drawn up the dining room table, to function as office desk, with a mess of papers, cuttings and documents — the counterpart to her obessive thoughts — filed in plastic shopping bags.

The settee where she slept had been pushed to one side. Her identification with the dead man surfaced when she mentioned that her husband had been in the habit of daytime dozing on the sofa, when he was on nightshift. Now it was littered with ashtrays, used crockery, dirty linen. A stale fug filled the house, an acrid fustiness that made breathing disagreeable. It was an effort to stay there, in that macabre house, with this lamentable woman whose wound would not heal.

I could think of nothing to break the impasse other than undertaking to visit her at intervals. I found the notion that she was identified with her dead husband interesting, if lurid, and a good starting point for an effort to make contact. I offered to come weekly, both to support her and in the hope that I might learn more about her state of mind.

One thing became clear: given time to talk to an interested listener, her conversation always turned to the question of the state of her husband's body after the impact. She had not been allowed to see the corpse, and she found this suspicious. The blood from her nose was repellent just because her husband's injuries then became more vivid. She was fixed in time, to the night of the accident, nearly two years ago, and in space to the trackside and the actions there of the flagman and her husband's mate. This man Ted, she was convinced had been negligent, and may have robbed the corpse of a pay pcket, as no money was found on the body.

After two or three weeks of this kind of talk, she fetched out from behind the sofa a paper carrier bulging with newspapers, solicitors' letters, insurance policies and correspondence, and invited me to look through them.

"They've offered me five thousand pounds compensation, but I won't accept. That isn't enough to compensate for a husband ..."

I found this unexpected. It was an undisputed and rational fact, I imagined, that she was entitled to compensation and that she should fight for the largest sum she could get. This was not in the least psychotic or spooky. On another visit I was astonished to learn that Ted, the alleged corpse robber, was a frequent visitor ....

Once, there was no answer to my knock, and I went away, mystified. That evening her neighbour, who after all continued to worry about her, rang me to say that Mrs Spriggs had been at home, but drunk: she had seen her through the window, "staggering about". The next day, when I went back, Mrs. Spriggs denied this, said she must have been asleep, then admitted she did occasionally have a drink to help get off. Who fetched it for her? Well, she did go out now and again to the local shops and to the post office for her pension. It had not occurred to me that she was capable of that: in all this time I had only seen her on her feet between the front door and her armchair. I decided to put some pressure on her to come down to the surgery once a week, rather than visit her.

She raised difficulties: she could walk short distances, but if she had to stand, she became dizzy, and whilst at the bus stop to the surgery there was a seat, there was none provided at the stop for the return journey. I countered with the idea that she might wait at her cousin's place, who lived very near the stop. She replied that her cousin's husband would not have her in the house. He was the one who had shouted at her *"why don't you kill yourself!"* and they were no longer on speaking terms.

125

I gave way, but next time she answered the door promptly, cigarette in mouth, but with a duster in her hand:

"I've been tidying up a bit, trying to tire myself out. I hoped I'd have heard from my sister in Brighton by now. I wrote to ask if I could stay with her for Christmas. Trouble is, last time I was there I took an overdose of my sleepers . . . "

I spoke to her a little about the phenomenon of her frightening people away, and the strangeness of the fact that her plight seemed soon to become unbearable to those who set out with good intentions. She looked at me, distrustfully, wondering if this was a criticism, but merely replied that if her sister failed her, she would prefer to spend Christmas in the psychiatric ward rather than be on her own. This was in October, but Christmas for her would be four days with the world closed down. I recalled my chilly wait on her doorstep in March, and imagined that in reverse: behind drawn curtains, doctors, social workers, neighbours, would drink and smoke their fill, and ignore her.

A Health Visitor, unknown to me, had befriended her and was also caught up in the impasse. She rang to ask whether I did not think Mrs Spriggs was best admitted to hospital, was it not dangerous for her to be at home alone, in that condition? I learned from her that Mrs Spriggs had arranged to hire a car, to be driven by Ted the suspected corpse robber, for the trip to her sister in Brighton, although it was clear that she was not wanted. I guessed the Health Visitor also now suffered from the toxic effect of Mrs Sprigg's state of mind, and felt her good intentions weighted down with dread.

I explained the difficulty with the hospital, her refusals and their reluctance, and my scepticism of its usefulness at present; I thought the problem was how to coax Mrs Spriggs from her refuge, that she took cover from her pain inside her lair, had found a partial sanctuary in the identification with her dead husband, but the subsequent impression she gave of being sorry for her self, rather than the victim, offended her friends. As an alternative initiative to the hospital, would she bring Mrs Spriggs to the surgery in her car, for a regular session of talk? She readily agreed.

Mrs Spriggs allowed the impasse to break, and submitted to

the combined persuasion of the Health Visitor and her cousin.
For the first time since the accident two years earlier she sat by
my desk. Her amiable escort consented to wait in the patients'
waiting room.

Mrs Spriggs, unsettled to find herself there, and feeling out-
manoeuvred, at first grumbled that the Health Visitor had
threatened her with hospital, then conceded that she was useful
for the collection of her pension from the post office.

She told me that she and Ted had in fact gone down to the
coast last week, and found no-one at home, but when I offered
a weekly discussion with me, she looked doubtful. She had been
unable to sleep wondering what I wanted. I talked to her of the
impression she gave me of being trapped "inside" the house,
inside a state of mind that she was unable to escape from. I tried
to convey to her my idea that she was a prisoner in a depression
that resembled her confused and neglected sitting room, that
the deadness of the room and of her mind was connected with
her husband's dead body. I reminded her of her remark to me
about the blood-stained paper tissues after her nose bleed, that
they made her picture her husband's injuries, and that she gave
the impression that she was identified with the dead body, as if
she couldn't be sure whether she was also a dead thing, or
trapped inside a dead body, unable to find a way out.

She listened to all this, sitting on the chair by the side of the
desk, a bemused frown on the squashed face, now turned to look
into mine. She answered with the comment that she had been
suspicious that I would have someone with me to force her into
a mental hospital, but that now she trusted me. She remembered when I came out at night once when she was ill, and how
her husband had always had faith in me. She relaxed her tense
position and smiled at me, a ray of warmth that I hadn't seen
from her before.

She accepted a small reduction in the dosage of her sedatives,
and agreed to come again in two weeks.

This next visit was a revelation. The intensity of her feeling
was awesome. She took me by surprise, frightened me a little
with an outburst from the depths. It was she who now demonstrated to me the mythical force of inner reality. She wept as she
described how she sensed the presence of her husband asleep on
the settee in the sitting room, or in his favourite armchair,

urging her to eat properly. She confessed she had at one time contemplated ending her own life as he had died, by throwing herself under a train.

She broke off, to collect herself, and mop her tears, then in a changed voice asked me to examine her left breast where she often felt a pain. I could find nothing wrong there, but was strengthened in the conviction that she had up to now been caught in an identification with the corpse of her dead husband.

I was moved by her declaration that he was sometimes alive and living in her mind. I said that in the life of the imagination it was possible for the dead to revive, and generate hopefulness and renewed interest in staying alive. If her husband remained a corpse in her mind she would feel dragged under by it, but it was evident that at present, this was not so, he was himself again, and concerned for her welfare; that this, merely in her imagination was not absurd, but of great significance for her recovery, and that these thoughts made it likely that the struggle to escape from her depression was now active in her mind.

I did my best to convey all this to her, while feeling uncertain of how much she understood, the concept of identification being so elusive and the crucial importance of the inner world of the imagination, a mysterious idea. But she had experienced some extraordinary mental states, and an actuality that corresponded either to what I was talking about, or if not, certainly to what I was doing.

As before, she responded indirectly by a warm smile and thanked me for the trouble I was taking with her.

The sympathetic Health Visitor brought Mrs Spriggs two weeks later. We talked again of the hallucinatory presence of her husband, real enough at times for her to reach out to him, while knowing there was nobody there. She told me that a date in January had been fixed by London Transport for the conclusion of the enquiry into the accident, and that Ted had been subpoenaed to appear.

Christmas panic was now escalating, a niece ceased to visit, the pain in her breast was troublesome, a nose bleed threatened, her fingers kept going .... dead! I called the psychiatrist to discuss a brief admission on compassionate grounds over the holiday period. His secretary rang back to say that the consultant

128

remembered Mrs Spriggs very well and was not prepared to admit her. He found her obstructive, and had warned her often that he would accept no further responsibility, until she was willing to help herself, particularly in the use of public transport.

I began to be aware that the buses were part of the same London Transport that was responsible for her husbands death.

I knew the consultant to be a hard man, but I assumed that this was unusual asperity even for him. Mrs Spriggs' uncanny capacity to make people fear and dislike her was, I think, evidence of the psychotic nature of her disturbance. I decided to speak to the consultant, in the hope that I could present her case more cogently. He was reluctant, said he would think about it and finally wrote to me:

> " . . . . if I receive a personal reassurance from you that she will be told that she has to find her own transport there and back, which she can well afford, and her alcohol consumption doesn't lead to inebriation, the only thing I am prepared to do is to allow her to come and have lunch here over the Christmas weekend . . . . "

His secretary read the letter to me over the phone before posting it. She then confessed that she had a similar one ready to send to Mrs Spriggs but had not the heart to send such a bad tempered letter, and had taken the responsibility of writing to her in more hospitable terms.

Mrs Spriggs and I met the requirements of the psychiatrist, and she survived Christmas. She began to eat more, and her weight increased. The offer of compensation from London Transport was improved to six thousand pounds, which she accepted. Her cramped, squashed features began to fill out, the ice was melting, and in our talks, now at monthly intervals, she wept more easily. The cousin who lived near the surgery, relieved that the ghoulish presence of the dead man had receded, shopped with her now only for food. The whisky she would have to fetch for herself.

Mrs Spriggs managed a visit on her own to the hairdresser, and commented that the traffic worried her, she didn't know why, because she wouldn't care that much if she got knocked down. But the mishap when it came was different.

There was a misunderstanding about an appointment: she came after I'd left, was offended, and missed her next one. I called on her, said that perhaps she felt I had lost interest in her. Cautiously, squinting at me through cigarette smoke, she nodded, but would not agree to visit me again. I decided to persist, and began to call again at intervals as before, hoping to regain the lost ground. She was unresponsive, sulky and unforgiving, and twice failed to answer my knock. I discovered that the Health Visitor who gave her a lift to the surgery, had left to get married and that her place had been taken by a psychiatric nurse, who roused her suspicions.

She would not budge on the question of visiting me, and I therefore continued my regular visits. Finally she melted again, and talked more explicitly about her thoughts, weeping as she did so.

"I want to die. I keep getting this picture in my mind of my husband being run over. I was getting a bit better I know, but now I feel very really bitter about them only giving me six thousand pounds. I think there must be a curse on every one connected with the accident, I've just heard that Ted has cancer now, and won't live long."

It was now over three years since the night of the accident. She felt always that he was on night shift, that she was waiting for him, and over and over again she saw the train strike him. My visits continued.

"Why did they send my cousin and me out of the court at the inquiry?" she ruminated a few months later. "They asked if my husband had any enemies! Well, that would have been manslaughter, wouldn't it? Ted's taken his secret to the grave, so I don't suppose the truth will ever come out. They told me I'd be able to see the body, but then they said it was better not to, because it was mutilated. What I can't make out is why they didn't want me to see it, I still think that if they'd both been killed together, Ted with him, it would make more sense."

A week or two later she responded to further discussion of the idea that she was trapped inside something, perhaps in imagination inside her husband's mutilated body:

130

"Is that why I feel both my legs are cut in two at the knee?"

She was developing painful swellings on the knee joints and the ankles, which quickly subsided with some tablets, but her movements were in general brisker, her glance softer. I sensed again a coming thaw. She arranged to take a summer holiday at the coast with her sister.

I called to see her in September on her return home.

"I seem to have got better!" she said opening the door with an embarrassed smile.

The windows were open, clean washing hung on the line, the sun lit up her sitting room. She was filled out and upright, had regained her former personality. She declared that for the first time in three and a half years she was feeling better. A few weeks later, she arrived at the surgery brought by a new Health Visitor. Now there was an excited note in her talk, and a gleam of triumph in her eye. I was anxious that she would tip over into a dangerous pseudo-cheerfulness. But the improvement was maintained as time passed. She reported that the thoughts were still there, but in the background. She was plagued by giddiness and sweating, and on the fourth anniversary of the accident, I was called to the house for a nose bleed.

Her thoughts were once more on the accident, and on other incidents to which she attached a morbid significance. A neighbour she disliked died, and a few months later his widow, whom she maintained had neglected her, was knocked down and killed by a van in the street. She began to have trouble with eczema. Then she stabilised, we agreed that she would contact me as required. Two years later, her cousin came into the surgery, and I realised I had no recent news of Mrs Spriggs. I learned that she was well, that they went out shopping together, but that she still slept on the couch in the sitting room, and avoided going upstairs.

Five years later, I received a similar answer . . . .

10   Born with the caul

Mrs Cole pulled a small suitcase from under the television table, and found amongst her papers and effects, a purse. In the purse was a silver snuff box. In the box, folded minutely, was a fragment of brown parchment, delicate and dry.

"I was born with the caul, you know that? I still have it here"

Her younger sister, an invalid confined to bed, exclaimed in surprise, and bent her neck to see. Mrs Cole was rightly confident of my interest in her exhibit — a portion of the amniotic membrane, preserved by her mother from the confinement in Bengal sixty years ago:

"Doctor, it means you'll be lucky you know. If a baby is born with the caul still round it, it's going to be a lucky baby, a good omen."

I looked it up later, in Brewer's dictionary, "a charm against death by drowning". Ellen Cole always knew what she was talking about. In fact, in the ordinary sense, she had not been very lucky, but she knew she was fortunate in her exceptionally sunny and affectionate temperament. That did preserve her from submersion by adversity both before and after she and her husband came to London from India.

She was about fifty when she first appeared at the surgery, cheerful and rotund: the chair creaked when she sat down. Her complexion was an alloy of metallic grey and pink tints, one part silver, three parts zinc, the hues soft, pearly, pastel.

Her lilting voice lifted and dipped, modulated in the Indian way. At our very first meeting, a complicated story was begun, which was to continue for years and years and which I never fully understood, because of the exuberance of her delivery, because many relatives and acquaintances, quite unknown to me of course, some still living in India, were confusingly referred to by their first names, but mainly because she was engaged in introducing me, bit by bit, into the complicated life of a being exceptionally gifted with a capacity for love.

133

The subtlety of her emotional life seemed to imply an identification with the railway system of the Indian subcontinent which she claimed was the oldest and most complex in Asia. The men in her family had worked on and with it for many generations, and it was inevitable that her marriage, when the time came, should be to a railway man. Mr Cole, to whom I was soon introduced, was a quiet man, ten years older than his wife. His benign nature complemented her exuberance, and he was content to allow her to do the talking.

Through the confusion of this first meeting, one item of information was delivered without ambiguity. I was to know that she had no live children — her four pregnancies had all been unsuccessful. Also that she was Catholic and European-Indian. She worked out her complicated descent for me later. Her father's grandfather was Armenian, his grandmother of mixed Irish and Spanish blood. On her mother's side also there were Catholics: Spanish and Irish forebears.

She was good tempered and humorous, but a persistent frequenter of the surgery. She suffered a little with wheezy bronchitis, but most of the consultations were about obesity, fluid retention, minor pains and swollen joints. Once she swelled to seventeen stone, but after strenuous efforts reduced to thirteen and a half. Her manner was eager, respectful, demure, and dignified by turns. On her right wrist she wore half a dozen thin gold bangles. Her umber eyes shone with valor, she wore her wavy hair short, eyebrows trimmed, plump cheeks touched with rouge, delicate mouth, straight nose, voice legato and piano. In summer, she wore a cotton dress open at the neck, exposing the foothills of a capacious bosom.

Her husband Albert, ex-Indian Railway foreman, worked on maintenance at the same factory where she was a coil winder. They put a deposit on a terrace house, and let the ground floor to distant relatives. They took immigrant status stoically, but at home in India, Mrs Cole sometimes wistfully reminded me, her parents had raised their two daughters in a spacious villa, with several servants and well stocked flower and kitchen gardens, two hundred miles from Calcutta. They attended a convent school to learn needlework, domestic science, and music. Nina, her sister went on to training college, became a kindergarten teacher, while Ellen helped her mother with the house, until her death at only forty five from an obscure infection. Ellen stayed on at home, looking after her father.

Then, she said, Nina made an unfortunate marriage, to a brute, a pig, who had insisted that all pregnancies be terminated, so that she could continue at work. Unbelievable villainy, a horrible man, so different, chalk and cheese, to industrious benevolent Albert, to whom Ellen was engaged. Their marriage took place after her younger sister's, but by then war had broken out in Europe, and life in India was changing for everyone.

After the war, and the death of her father, came the partition of India. Many Anglo-Indian friends came to England. As Catholics they felt that war between Hindu and Muslim was one they had best avoid. They hesitated, Nina would be left behind with that horror of a husband, who was now totally neglecting her since she had become lame in one leg. There was nothing they could do about it.

They were not lonely here, Mrs Cole was gregarious, they were both industrious and prudent. For all its difference from the villa in Bengal, their upstairs flat in London N.W. was a useful base from which to establish new friendships. Next door, Mrs Connolly and her five beautiful children were soon on intimate terms, old Mr Birch that recalcitrant widower, who trundled a two wheeled cart about the streets with his decorator's equipment, was induced to give up his insularity and benefit from Mrs Cole's buxom warmth, and Miss Kerr, the eccentric cat lover two doors away, found a new ally.

The character of local shopkeepers and the quality of their merchandise, having been assessed, those she patronised recognised in her a good customer, but a canny shopper. She bought only the best quality fruit and vegetables, and her domestic economy was fine-tuned. She became close friends with an Anglo-Indian lady of considerable beauty, who had married an Englishman with no business capacity. Their shop sold Indian brass and leather goods and stuffs and materials for dressmaking. Mrs Cole, out of sympathy with her friend, after long discussions behind the counter on her domestic problems, bought material she didn't need and then made it up into aprons, or tea cloths, or other items for distribution to her friends.

The local priest called occasionally, but for all her conscious-
ness of Catholicism, Mrs Cole was by nature a free spirit.
Religion was part of her childhood culture, acknowledged with
filial respect, but when it came to the realities of the world, she
needed no other divine inspiration than that which she found
within. Her natural generosity enabled her to think clearly
about the behaviour and character of others and thus navigate
herself and her husband through the shark infested waters of
large organisations, including the medical and clerical.

Nina was spoken of more and more as time passed. She had
a mysterious illness: a limp first, in her thirties, then difficulty
with speech and vision. Nothing could be done for her in India,
her husband would not pay. One day they would bring her to
London. Mrs Cole spoke with such venom about her brother-
in-law, I wondered what had attracted her sister to him: he was
very handsome, she shrugged. Then one day: triumph! *The pig
was dead*. Mrs Cole's satisfaction was great, except that her
sister now lay neglected in a pauper hospital for incurable
diseases in a backwater of rural India. She was leaving for
India to fetch the invalid home, and hoped I would help them
to care for her.

My first sight of Nina was a ponderous five foot nine figure of
sixteen stone, who ranged with elephantine momentum from
one support to another, chair-arm to table, around the upstairs
flat living room, like a wounded creature from the wild: spastic
muscles swung bulky limbs wide to clear the carpet. Much taller
than Ellen, her grey metallic complexion was similar, but her
gaze had the mildness suited to a kindergarten teacher. She
goggled through spectacles, with eyes more round, more liquid,
than her older sister's, as squint and nystagmus betrayed the
illness that attacked her: multiple sclerosis.

Together, the sisters filled up the small room, and buzzed
with the excitement of the reunion. Mr Cole presided calmly,
over this permanent alteration to his domestic arrangements. I
never heard him complain as the invalid became central to their
lives. But the tenants of the downstairs flat felt the change. This
unfortunate complacent couple were at first determined not to
move, whatever inducement or threat was offered. But a mysterious force came to Mrs Cole's aid. Padre Pio, of Pitrelcina,
was a Catholic priest. When, in 1918, "the Five Wounds of Our

Lord's Passion" appeared on his body, making him the first priest with the stigmata in the history of the Church, he attracted world wide attention, according to the Coles, who were his devoted admirers. His picture hung on the wall, next to a large tapestry of The Last Supper. Both ladies wore amulets with his potrait at their wrists and throats. Mr Cole was despatched on a pilgrimage to Italy. On his return, Mrs Cole was triumphant.

"Doctor, Padre Pio read Albert's thoughts! As soon as he came home those people downstairs told me they had decided to leave! He wanted a hundred pounds, but I said we hadn't asked him to go. You see, I'm not stupid! He came down to sixty, but what d'you think, doctor, he called Albert a bastard! Terrible, eh? These people have no respect for their fathers. I said he must be Albert's father himself . . . ."

She shook with amusement at her own audacity.

The house was reorganised, the front room downstairs became Nina's bed sitting room. The fireplace was boarded up, storage heaters installed; Mr Cole re-decorated: lemon wallpaper and white woodwork; furniture: a bed and an armchair for Nina, an immense sofa as a general repository for clean linen, clothes, blankets, household effects — and for Ellen to sleep on if night supervision was needed. The items which collected on mantelpieces everywhere, here included a large plaster Madonna and child, and a smaller black priest holding a prayer book, and a picture of Padre Pio brought back by Albert from Italy. A twenty inch colour TV commanded a corner, its table handy for tablets and other medical supplies. Faded black and white studio portraits of the ladies' mother and father, looking serious in a Calcutta studio, hung by the fireplace with a colour picture of Pope John, smiling benignly. Surprisingly, a photograph of a moustached, complacent, handsome man, was also affixed to the wall. Nina could contemplate this image of her late husband at her leisure.

In this room, where Mrs Cole and I conferred so often over Nina, as she became confined to bed, I would persuade her to talk about her life before the partition of India, and the decision to emigrate to England.

It was not just curiosity. Mrs Cole was an engrossing talker, but she needed encouragement to start and prompting to

137

continue: she was not one to talk much about herself, except when her feelings overflowed. The thread of her narrative often tangled, and after several years of entranced listening I was too embarrassed to admit that all was not clear. Her mind was furnished with reflections on many curious experiences and anecdotes. There was naive religious piety from her childhood, blended with a capacity for thought and attention to reality which was the very opposite of superstition. Her childlessness was tragic, the history of her miscarriages bizarre. She was authoritative and generous, courageous and humorous, calm and impatient of cant: a natural leader but with only a small band of followers: her husband, her sister, some friends.

"Our home was near Calcutta, doctor. Our father, a fine looking man, was educated at a convent school — we are Catholics you know that. When he was still young, his mother started thinking about finding a suitable bride for him. She heard of a girl in Bombay and went to visit her home there. The girl was only fifteen, and her father had died of Asian cholera. D'you know about the Asian cholera, Doctor? It turns you black! Grandmother said to the girl's mother 'I would like to take her home with me'. It's a long way you know, Bombay to Calcutta, it's nearly two thousand miles. At sixteen she married my father. Once, when she was pregnant with me, she was on the veranda, when a lizard jumped down her chest. For that reason I've always been frightened of them. One lived in the bathroom above the water cistern. Before I had a bath I had to call the servant, 'Is it there?' 'Yes, memsahib, I will remove it.' You know doctor, my mother was just seventeen, when I was born — with the caul."

This was the time she pulled out the suitcase to show me the caul.

"We had a lovely home, doctor. On Sundays, fifty beggars would come and wait under the tamarind tree at the bottom of the garden, holding their gourds, and crying out "Oh, Mamma," Mother would go round using father's Wills' cigarette tobacco tin to measure out rice and dahl from big baskets carried by servants, and give each one of them sixpence."

"Oh Mamma" Nina suddenly sang out, "Oh Mamma!" She was in her hammock, suspended from a hydraulic lift, her alternative to bed. She had followed the story with glistening eyes from which a tear now trickled. She spoke so little and with such difficulty at this time, that her presence, like that of a silent child, might be temporarily overlooked.

Mrs Cole eyed her with a mixture of amusement, pride and pain.

"That was a lovely house, you know, doctor, the station master's house by the river, in Bihar. In the summer you could wade across to the other side, but in the monsoon it was like an impassable wall of water. Our neighbour, Mr Bhose was a horticulturist: he had a wonderful garden and sent mother a basket of flowers every Sunday. You should go to India, doctor. You'd be a millionaire! But you'd have to stipulate private practice, money paid in sterling U.K. You must know about" (she began to tick them off on her fingers), cholera, typhoid, chickenpox, smallpox, beri-beri and malaria. You'd be a millionaire in no time."

Mr Cole smiled his assent. He enjoyed his wife's dramaturgy, and chipped in with supplementary information: he had heard all her stories before, and enjoyed them more with each telling. After sixty five, retired from the shop floor, he was re-employed as a security guard, and, he said, was so highly regarded in this post, that he was immediately promoted to the top and rewarded with generous bonuses at every opportunity. His flair in security must have come from his managerial skills, for his physique, unlike that of his wife and sister-in-law, was not on the grand scale.

He was ten years older than Mrs Cole, who was proud of his vitality, reliability, and satisfaction with her domestic provision; he submitted happily to the matriarchal atmosphere of the home. Beaming through elegant spectacles, he complemented his wife's buxom forthrightness with a feminine delicacy of manner. There was a clerical air about his smooth brow and mild countenance. He rarely looked worried, except when plagued by a runny nose: this brought him to the surgery in a panic, which only responded to the most vehement of reassurance. He told me that his mother died from a snake bite

139

when he was six, no doubt this contributed to his lack of self confidence in health matters. He was the third of four sons of a regular soldier, who sent each boy in their turn to a military school in Calcutta. Later, he worked as a fireman on the railway, and progressed to responsibility for an engine shed. His father was killed in 1942 at the North West Frontier.

He and Ellen were married soon after the war began, when she was thirty, and he was forty.

The story of Ellen's four failed pregnancies, was peculiar, and it was only gradually that I was able to make out what had happened. She had followed her husband to his wartime postings. In 1943 he was involved in the railway preparations for the invasion of Burma. She told me that after the victory of the Eighth Army in North Africa, it was reconstituted in Eastern India as the Fourteenth Army and acted in conjunction with American troops in eastern India. Railway workers were encamped in the forest with their families, and liaised with army transport. Accommodation was in wooden huts, overrun at night by rats, scorpions and snakes. Their human neighbours too, were unattractive: the local brothels were kept busy.

"You know, doctor, the Americans released criminals from Sing Sing on condition they went into the front line on the advance into Burma! We were surrounded on all sides by these terrible people. It was only because the legs of the beds were slippery that we were protected from all the snakes. That was a terrible place: if a Chinese servant came into an army tent and took a cigarette, he had to kneel down and was shot on the spot.

I was just married you know. We didn't know much about birth control . . . in that horrible place . . . I was pregnant four times . . . I lost all my babies, stillborn, but the fourth time, that was the worst . . . when I went into labour, they sent for the doctor . . . it was a long way, a long time before he came . . . before he arrived the baby . . . was there . . . as I sat on the commode . . . an Indian doctor . . . You know, some of those Indian doctors in those days . . . I don't think he was a proper doctor. He kept crystals of bromide in his top pocket . . . took them all the time he spoke to you . . . prescribed them for his patients and then took some himself.

Conditions there were terrible ... septicaemia set in ... I was an emergency case. I was taken by ambulance to the American Army hospital ... a lovely surgeon saved my life .... Mr MacDonald, I'll never forget him."

Her religious enthusiasm was not indiscrimate:

"You know, doctor, the worst priests in India are Jesuits. They know all the theory, but I know it here in the heart from practical suffering. I had four baby boys, all stillborn. When I held them in my arms and cried, that was real feeling. Priests can be bigoted, you know that? Jesus didn't invent religion, all He said was 'Love thy neighbour'. Man invented religion, all those different ones – and then they squabble with one another about it."

A few years later — these conversations were continued over long periods of time — I heard a sequel:

"When my first baby was stillborn, I wanted my father to see it. I put it's little body in a bottle with spirit to preserve it, until he could come and visit us. He was very upset, when he saw it, told me I shouldn't have, so then I arranged for it to be buried. You know, after that last baby I told you about, and the big operation at the American Hospital? After the war we were back home again and I was sitting on the veranda weeping. A servant girl from the villa next door asked me what was the matter. I told her I didn't want any more pregnancies. She arranged for the village midwife to come to me. She asked me when my next period would be, and when the time came, she took some white powder, mixed it with a little milk, heated it on the stove, then gave it to me to drink. Doctor, if quinine is bitter, this was the grandfather of quinine. She gave me this thing for the next two periods and after that I never became pregnant again."

The Coles were able to realise their frustrated capacity for care with Nina. Mrs Cole also had her "daughters": two excitable silky terriers, not more than eight inches high, who rushed yelping to the front door, in response to the bell. They leaped and yapped, demanding attention until offered a cheek to kiss, which they did from their "mother's" arms, with a gentle lick, after which they subsided beneath the sofa, and watched the rest of the consultation from there. When Mr Cole was expected, they took up position on Nina's bedhead, from where they could see the garden gate. They waited quietly until he appeared, then flung themselves out to the hall and the front door for the kiss. They were mother and daughter — it was a sad day when the daughter was run over and killed in the road.

Then there was Barbara, the child of friends from India. She was in fact the youngest of three children, whose mother had died when Barbara was about six. They lived outside London, but Mrs Cole wrote to her every week and enclosed a postal order. Barbara wrote back each week, with news of the family and her school progress. At first these were childish scribbles enclosed in letters from her father, but as time passed her letters became more mature and meaningful. Mrs Cole showed me an extra letter from eleven year old Barbara, which she considered pure intuition, as Albert, nearing eighty was in hospital for suspected lung cancer.

"Dear Aunt Ellen" the letter began, "Do not reply to this letter seeing it's an extra one . . . . "

At Christmas the three children and their father came to stay. He had trained for the priesthood until he fell in love and married. He was a tall slim, gently spoken man, with a melancholy air, whom I met several times there. He was I think a little embarrassed by his family's neediness at Christmas and by his indebtedness to the Coles. Christmas was a large occasion in that house, and food and gifts were always provided for my family, with coins hidden amongst the sweets for the children. I felt that Barbara and Mrs Cole were well matched and lucky to have one another, the one finding a mother, the other a daughter.

When Barbara reached adolescence, she gave her father a difficult time with her boy friends, described at third hand to me as wild and crude. Her father wrote to the Coles of his anxiety about her, and his anguish at the absence of a mother who might have helped Barbara. Mrs Cole from eighty miles away, was at a loss, and tried her best to influence Barbara in her letters. When this failed and it was clear that Barbara would go her own way, Mrs Cole found it impossible to avoid an increasingly reproachful tone, both to Barbara, and to her father whose efforts to control his daughter she thought weak and inadequate. The relationship between the two families broke down. Like many good and well intentioned people, Mrs Cole although full of human kindness and altruism, found the anarchy of adolescence beyond her capacity to bear.

The situation grew worse. the name of one boy friend emerged from the pack; and in the version I was hearing, he did not sound promising, being unemployed, uneducated, and without talent for anything but taking advantage of a vulnerable girl without a mother. At seventeen Barbara was reported pregnant, and then married. Mrs Cole struggled with her feelings. She sent some baby clothes, and showed me some photographs, but she was hurt. In any case it was now clear that Albert was not going to survive much longer — there were two invalids to worry about.

Now, I called there at regular intervals. Once she handed me a little coloured card,

"Take this little prayer, doctor. Always carry it with you. It will help you in your work. I wear mine in my bra!"

I slipped it into my pad of papers, and found it there many years later:

A Physician's Prayer

Lord, Thou Great Physician,
I kneel before thee. Since
every good and perfect gift
must come from Thee,

I PRAY
Give skill to my hand, clear
vision to my mind, kindness
and sympathy to my heart.
Give me singleness of pur-
pose, strength to lift at least
a part of the burden of my
suffering fellowmen, and a
true realisation of the rare

> *privilege that is mine, Take*
> *from my heart all guile and*
> *worldliness, that with the*
> *simple faith of a child I may*
> *rely on Thee. Amen.*

After fourteen years of caring for her sister, Mrs Cole's task had become much heavier and absorbed most of her energy. Once she retired from work, she rarely left the house other than to shop, or for her weekly hair appointment. On two occasions, Nina was admitted to a geriatric ward, to allow the Coles a fortnight's holiday. Each time she was delivered home with bed sores: no more holidays were taken after this. The next hospital admission was an emergency for an abscess around the kidney.

Nina was home again two weeks later: I found Mrs Cole bending over her sister's flank, poking ribbon gauze into the wound in her side, with the aplomb of an experienced nurse.

"I should have been a Matron, doctor. My father was a medical student in India. One day he had to watch a leg being amputated. He didn't stop running!"

Mr Cole who watched his wife with admiration added,

"When I worked in the engine sheds I often saw coolies legs cut off in railway accidents. Those Hindu coolies worked in the shunting yards shovelling coal, and sometimes they fell asleep on the line — there were terrible accidents. Hindus won't touch a dead body, you know. I was the one always called to do it."

"It's true, doctor," added his wife, as she carefully applied a dressing to the packed wound, "sometimes he would come home after an accident and wouldn't touch his dinner . . . ."

A few days later I found her in mock ill humour.

"Nina will only say 'yes' and 'no' today. Shall I kill her, doctor?"

But Nina's taciturnity was due to a fever, she was building up another abscess in her loin and was admitted to hospital again, for removal of the kidney. Mrs Cole telephoned after the operation.

144

"I spoke to the surgeon, a very nice man, Portuguese I think, his name is Rubello. I said to him, 'I hope you are clever'" (mocking her own coyness) "I said it straight to him you know, and he smiled and said there was seventy per cent chance of success. I said I would pray God should move his hands in the right direction. They are going to do it at four, at the end of the list, because of all that dirty pus flying about. Pray for Nina tomorrow doctor, between four and six."

Another call came from her the next evening,

"That kidney was useless to her! She had a big stone there. I said to the Sister 'Have you given Nina's kidney a Catholic burial?' She didn't know whether I was joking!"

Nina survived the operation and life went on in the front room as before, even after the death of Albert. Sometimes Mrs Cole was ready with conversation and reminiscences, at other times she was weighed down by the restricted life she was leading and the total absorption in her patient.

On one occasion, having told me quietly about some news from Barbara's father, and commented on how the talks we had together helped her to get things off her chest, so that she didn't feel choked by them, she put her hand on my shoulder as we stood by Nina's bedside:

"You know, doctor, I wish you were my brother. We never had a brother, but I love you as if you were." She frowned a little, embarrassed. "It's nothing sexual, you know, some people do feel like that with their doctors, you know that. Just like brother and sister . . . ."

11   Group Discussion

The members of the group:

Conrad. Shall I start? Now we've all read each other's stories, what's the general opinion? What do you all think?

Jim. He always was difficult to follow, but he did try. My Mum thought he was a good doctor.

Mrs Wall. I went to see him after my first breakdown, and I liked talking to him, but my Fred got suspicious. He was a bit like you Roy, he thought it was all rubbish, said he'd get himself into trouble one day putting everything down to nerves.

Mrs Spriggs. Don't talk to me about nerves. That horrible psychiatrist, did you see what he wrote about me?

Mrs Cole. I don't know anything about nerves, that's one thing my family never suffered from. Look what Nina went through, that was enough to give anyone a nervous break-down, that was real suffering, not just the imagination . . .

Henry Lake. They say it's worse when it's in the mind. I had something on my mind about Sheila, my ex-wife. I thought I wasn't that kiddy's father, but she said I was imagining it.

Jim. My Mum used to imagine that our Dad was having an affair with someone else.

Roy. What about when I got stuck in that lay-by. I said I felt

147

boxed-in. I never could understand why, when I asked him why my nerves affect what I love most, cars, he said they were my parents.

Ghost of Fred Wall. Seems to me the doctor got on better with the ladies than with us men, wouldn't you say Mr Lake?

Henry Lake. I used to think he took my wife's side, and I'm sure he had something to do with us losing the house, and Ann suddenly being difficult to live with. I think its the sex thing. I remember when he first came to that practice. He was quite good then, delivered one of my kids. But when he got older he couldn't be bothered so much, told my mother she had asthma, when it was cancer.

Ghost of Mr Wall. I fooled him that way, had a good laugh afterwards. Wish I'd been there to see his face.

Mrs Wall. That wasn't his fault, he told you to rest and you wouldn't do it. You wanted to die, you know you did. That was your way of spiting me.

Mrs E Cook. If that's true I hope he's ashamed of himself wherever he is. We don't hold . . .

Mrs D Cook. . . . with that sort of thing. It's sheer cowardice. Look at what I've been through. I had TB same as him, and psoriasis, and a prolapse.

Mr Rogers. I was certainly ashamed of myself, after I tried to kill myself on the beach. I don't know really why I did it. I don't think it was because of the girl. He said it had something to do with the death of my father the year before, but I never really felt I knew what he was getting at.

Mrs Wall. He scared me. I was sure he would put all my pains down to nerves, and I'd find I had cancer.

Ghost of Mr Wall. He definitely told me the pain was in my mind. Definitely. As a matter of fact, it might be actionable.

Ann Lake. I've had a look at that story about us. It's true, the hospital did keep changing their minds about mother-in-law's asthma. It was they who said it wasn't cancer in the first place, and I'm glad they did. It was better for her not to know.

Mrs E Cook. He came to see me in hospital after my big operation. I see he's had his bit of fun with us about him being a clean doctor and all that, but one thing . . . .

Mrs D Cook. ... we won't put up with is slovenliness. Mrs Spriggs, – o' course we're very sorry about Mr Spriggs, and if you'd lived a bit nearer, we would have tried to help you, – but to let yourself go like that, and let it get on top of you, that's what we can't understand. Why don't people be like us, and take ...

Mrs E Cook. ... their minds off their troubles by keeping themselves busy. There's never a moment when Dora and I aren't dusting, cleaning, washing, baking.

Mrs Cole. I noticed in your story ladies, that you baked for him like me. He did well, getting it from both of us.

Mr Rogers. Cake or no cake, I've nothing against the man. I have to say that he helped me quite a bit when I was really down. I .... well of course a father's a father, I'd like to think my kids would spare a thought for me. All that about the evacuees, that surprised me, I haven't thought about that for years. I wonder if it was talking about that brought the eczema back. He rather wanted me to think it was because he went on holiday, and of course I did have a bad spell of it after my father died, shingles, skin cancer ...

Conrad. See page 8, the protomental.

Mr Rogers. I dismiss all that.

Jim. I was interested in that bit, 'e said my troubles started when I was a nipper too, and I was never much good at thinkin'. They thought I was backward, and I never learned to read and write what you would call properly, but if I 'ad a father like him, I might even 'ave been a doctor! I asked my Mum about it, she didn't see what that 'ad to do with it, I was all right really 'til I broke my leg.

Mrs E Cook. Your trouble, young man, was drinking all that cider and getting addicted to all those horrible tranquilisers.

Conrad. Yes, but the point is, that's how his parents were. That's the identification. Now my father before the war was a headmaster. Horrible to think that he ended up like a smelly old tramp. You'd never recognise him as the man he was. Chalk and cheese.

Ghost of Mr. Wall. He'd say faeces and nipple most likely.

Mrs Cole. My father didn't deteriorate, I'm relieved to say. He was the same dignified stationmaster right to the end of the line.

Henry Lake. I thought you went in for that Padre?

Mrs Cole. Padre Pio had the stigmata. It symbolised his suffering on behalf of us all — his identification with Jesus, about His Father's business.

Roy. My Dad's is a garage business, like his father before him.

Conrad. The family business. Stepping into father's shoes, I understand that better now. He says that he thought I ought to have moved out of the ground floor flat and let my parents have it, but my mother was very stubborn. Once she got an idea into her head, nothing could shift it. That's why I could never talk to them about my problems, they used to worry about me so much. But things get clearer with experience. It's all to do with who you are. My first wife didn't want to be Polish, she wanted to be British. What did she do? She played a trick on me, got inside my life on false pretences. That's what he means by the car, Roy. It's like dressing up as someone you're not, then you get trapped inside there and can't get out. In your mind that is, although people do it for real too . . .

Roy. Sorry I just don't see it. And if it's my mind doing it I'd rather hit it with anti-depressants. I never want to go through that again. Or the shock treatment.

Ann Lake. The amount of valium I took frightened my mother. She blamed the doctors for giving them out too easily, but if you're like I was there's no way you're going to manage without them.

Jim. One time I was gettin' 'em from both the psychiatrist and from 'im. 'E'd been tryin' to cut me down, so I told a lie and got a second supply from the 'ospital. Then they got in touch with one another, and after that . . . .

Conrad. Yes, this question of the doctors getting together to discuss us . . . . Are we to consider it as being an advantage, two heads better than one, or as a breach of confidence? It has its advantages and disadvantages. For example, is Jim here better off because his supply of drugs was cut down, or has he a grumble because can't get as many as he wants?

Mrs Wall. After I took my overdose, he stopped giving them to me altogether. I used to beg him just to give me enough to get a decent night's sleep, that he could trust me. That reminds me, it was so embarrassing when I said I could trust him without a chaperone and he said he couldn't trust me. I blushed.

Conrad. He was trying to psycho-analyse us. Turning things round the wrong way, or the right way, it all depends on the way you think about it.

Ghost of Mr Wall. That's what I think. An amateur psychiatrist.

Conrad. No, no, it's psycho-analysis. Freud, Klein and Bion. It's all there in Chapter One. I could see at the end he wanted to prove to me that I was suffering from an Oedipus Complex, that I wanted to get rid of Dad.

Mrs D. Cook. He would never say a thing like that, he was the soul of kindness to me and my Jim . . . .

Conrad. Look, it's not a question of him saying it. You remember how he starts my story, puts down something about my going to see him, it's all rather personal, I don't want to discuss that. But I went to this clinic, and that's where they talk to you about the Oedipus Complex. Girls and their fathers . . .

Mrs Cole. Papa I called mine. Like the Pope. I always kept a picture of him near Nina, next to one of Padre Pio. I thought Doctor looked like Pope John. I told him once — I was very upset at the time — that I loved him like a brother. Then, I felt a bit shy, I went and said that it wasn't anything sexual. If he's psycho-analysing us . . .

Ann Lake. I think he fell in love with me a bit at the end, just the way he smiled at me. Probably I'm just imagining it.

Henry Lake. "Just" imagining it!

Conrad. Yes, good point. How about saying, it doesn't matter it's just real? That's the attitude of some of these psycho-analysts.

Ann Lake. I used to worry a bit about him, thought he looked a bit tired. I don't think he liked being called out on his half day . . .

Conrad. Yes that's what I mean, that's what's supposed to happen with women . . .

Mrs Spriggs. I never had time for anyone but my Bill. Now the sooner I drink and smoke myself out of it the better.

Mrs Wall. Smoking can damage your health.

Ghost of Mr Wall. Yes, and so can doctors, some of them.

Henry Lake. Hold on. Doesn't he imply in Mrs Spriggs' story that he cured her? Doesn't sound cured to me.

151

Conrad. My point is that these psycho-analysts don't take account of what's happened to you in real life. It's all related to the imagination, and everyone's life is so different. Frankly, with respect, none of you really know what real fear is.If you'd lived through what we had to, the Germans coming at us one way, and when we tried to get away, we met people running towards us and away from the Russians. Father was in prison, could have been shot, all of us in Siberia, then across Russia, the Middle East, India ... can't understand you English. I mean with all due respect to you, sir, separated from your Mummy and Daddy and going to pieces! To be truthful I have tried to understand Chapter One. The bit about the old lady at the end of course that's interesting. I know he liked talking to old ladies, my mother had the highest opinion of him, but personally I think he had an Oedipus Complex himself.

Roy. I don't concentrate very well when it comes to reading books. But with cars, I can get through with a manual, no problem ....

Ghost of Mr Wall. (*sotto voice*). Wanker!

Roy .... so how d'you explain that? Anyway, if you've read it and tell me it's rubbish that won't surprise me.

Jim. My readin's not very good, but there was a bit there about pain, I see 'e's put in what I wrote that time, and called it a poem, that's funny, me writin' poetry, and 'e's put in a couple of my dreams, about bein' a baby, stuff comin' out of me mouth and behind, it's a bit embarrassin' ...

Conrad. That's where the bit about spilling out of the container comes in I expect.

Mr Rogers. And he's got one of his own dreams in. Should he be telling us about himself? That bit about him when he was a boy, that surprised me. Aren't they not supposed to tell you anything about themselves ....

Conrad. Counter-transference. I think he was identified with you.

Mrs Wall. I see he's put in my dreams about Fred trying to pull me after him. But I've stopped reading too now, haven't got the patience, not even for the newspaper. When my Fred was alive he used to read the Sporting Pink. Probably don't do it any more since the war.

Ghost of Mr Wall. Sporting Pink? We still get it down here.

Mrs Wall. Everything's changed since we were children, the world's a different place. I put it down to the war. Have you noticed how many of you talk about the war, Jim and the bombs, I lived through that too, the Polish gentleman here, Mr Rogers, Mrs Cole. They say Hitler was mad. Why d'you think nobody stopped him, before it was too late?

Mrs Spriggs. I did war work – did you notice that bit about me running for cover when they strafed the factory? But I'd like to ask your late husband a question, Mrs Wall. You didn't hear any news of my husband, Mr. William George Spriggs, about five nine, eleven stone, clean shaven, pleasant look about him – course that was before he was hit by the train? But I've heard that makes no difference afterwards, if you've lived a good life, you get repaired to how you were before the accident, a sort of miracle.

Conrad. That's in the imagination. You're confusing external and internal reality. That's what the problem was with Hitler. Everyone thought it must be a bad dream.

Ghost of Mr Wall. Mrs Spriggs, don't you worry, my dear. I've had a quick read of your story. He's gone, you know, the other place, where good people go, not devils like me, eh Gloria?

Mrs Wall. Is the poodle with you? I don't know why I had her put down. I must have been mad. She was our baby, kind of symbolic.

Mrs Cole. Life after death? That's what the Jesuits used to tell us, and when I was a little girl in Bihar, we believed it. But now I think everyone makes their own heaven and hell.

Roy. I don't get you lot, if ever I get out of this box, symbolic or not, imaginary or not . . . .

Mrs Cole. That's your hell, Roy.

Roy. But I didn't make it myself. And my idea of heaven is a Lamborghini. Dad'll help.

Conrad. Now I understand why he said your car was your mother.

Mrs E Cook. Roy, I've just had a look at your story and I think its pathetic. I really don't know whether to laugh or cry. That bit about your father coming home without the baby, and you saying "where's the baby? In the suitcase?" '

153

Henry Lake. Yes, and then you saying you felt you were shut up in a box yourself! So you're the same as the baby!

Conrad. "The same as" . . . there's that bit about Jim damaging his left leg, the same as his father.

Mr Rogers. And Mrs Spriggs here, same as her poor Bill, all that blood and "both legs cut off below the knee".

Mrs Spriggs. But that was only in my imagination! . . . . Oh dear, yes, I see. But aren't medical notes supposed to be confidential? I don't like the idea of everyone reading about my private life.

Mrs D Cook. It's to help others. It's only fair if you're being helped yourself . . .

Mrs Ann Lake. I'm a bit worried about the confidentiality. After all, he does rather suggest that there was something a bit, well, perverted about me putting up with Henry here for so long.

Conrad. Masochism!

Mrs Wall. If anyone was a masochist, I was. Why I put up with Fred for so long, I don't know. But what could I do? He was ill and nobody would look after him if I didn't. His sisters left it all to me.

Henry Lake. Perverted? Did he say that?

Mrs Lake. No, course he didn't say so. Not in so many words. But he kind of suggested it.

Conrad. Sometimes I think they're all homo's themselves.

Mr Rogers. No, it's not that. This sexual thing goes very deep. I mean, look at young Roy here. Why should he have a breakdown just when he's become engaged? Look at me, how I went off the rails, and why? The girl meant nothing to me.

Mrs Wall. Sex, and jealousy, that's what was the undoing of my marriage. My Fred was so suspicious. Well, I have admitted I started it, I used to make him jealous, but then he got his own back, I used to look on his coat for other women's hairs — and I found one once!

Conrad. Hair splitting — and projective identification! Folie a deux! Voyeurism! Sado masochism!

Jim. I'll 'ave to look those up in me Dad's dictionary when I get 'ome.

Mrs Wall. You won't be any the wiser. You've got to experience it, to understand it. The thing I don't understand is how they can tell the difference between pain when you're really ill, cancer say, and when you're imagining it .... well, when it's in your mind anyway.

Jim. That was funny, when 'e said I was gettin' labour pains!

Henry Lake. They *must* have been imaginary.

Conrad. Identified with a woman in labour, you think?

Roy. Well, its obvious that most of us are here because we've had breakdowns, but what about these two ladies, and Mrs Cole? They've never been anywhere near a psychiatrist. What are they doing here? All I'm saying is, you three aren't nerve cases like the rest of us. And I assume *he's* never had a nervous breakdown. What I want to know is how can someone who hasn't been through it, hasn't experienced it, understand what it's like?

Mr Rogers. We've all been through it in our own way.

Mrs Cole. These ladies are here for the same reason as me.

Mrs E Cook. Yes. Life is more than being ill and miserable, there has to be someone well enough to look after the sick.

Mrs D Cook. I never asked anyone for sympathy in all my life. Not even when I was strapped to a board in the TB hospital for six months. I never had any children myself, Roy, but I think that the way you treat your father and mother, well I know my Jim never put up with that from Brian ....

Mr Rogers. He still gave you a lot of worry.

Mrs Spriggs. My Bill and I never had any children either.

Mrs Wall. And neither did I.

Mrs Cole. And Nina and I lost all ours.

Conrad. Let's change the subject. What d'you all ....

Mrs Lake. Hold on. Why d'you want to change the subject? I think it's a very important one. Sometimes I think you men have no idea what it means to a woman, to bear a child and have the responsibility for it for the rest of your life.

Mr Rogers. Are you a feminist, then?

Mrs Lake. Not exactly. But how can a man know what it's like to have a baby at the breast? The uncertainty can be terrible. Sometimes I felt I wanted to suckle more than he wanted to suck, at other times I was worried sick. In the end I had to wean him early, I couldn't stand the worry that he wasn't getting enough nourishment.

Roy. Poor little sod!

155

Mr Rogers. I think it's more the difference between grown ups and children, than men and women. Fathers can take responsibility for looking after children. But children can't look after themselves for long without getting into trouble or running into danger, or feeling ill.

Conrad. Stiff necks. They worship false gods like Baal-zebub, The Lord of the Flies. Which reminds me I was going to say what do you think of the way he puts down things that we wrote? He's got Jim's "poem" and my "Brief Mental History ..."

Mrs Spriggs. And even my letter ...

Conrad. .... not to mention "The Physician's Prayer".

Ghost of Mr Wall. .... Which this good lady here kept in her bra, ha, ha.

Mrs Cole. Yes, and that's just what he says, doesn't he in Chapter One. I've read it, all that about the breast and the ... and the nipple.

Conrad. Introjective Identification? I'm still worried about the question of confidentiality.

Ghost of Mr Wall. And me about calling every pain imaginary ....

Mrs Cole. And me about how I'll end up now I've lost my husband and my sister. But God will provide for me, like I provided for Nina.

The Mrs Cooks. We never worry, let every day take care of itself, that's our motto ...

A disembodied voice. Time's up, I'm afraid.

Roy. I was just beginning to enjoy it. I think I'll stay on a bit, it looks cold outside. (*Looks round anxiously, after a minute*). Who's there? I thought I heard a funny noise. Oh, it's you Dad. I didn't know you came here. I seem to have got left behind, and don't know the way out. Can you show me how it's done? ....

Kennith Sanders   -   NINE LIVES:
                        THE EMOTIONAL EXPERIENCE IN GENERAL PRACTICE
                        (Clunie Press   1991)

This is an unusual book by an unusual person - a general
practitioner, trained as a psychoanalyst, working as a general
practitioner. It chronicles his experiences as a principal in a
busy general practice, in a depressed part of North West London,
over thirty years. To do so the author chooses the lives of nine
ordinary people and their families and describes the many and
various ways they used him in his role as "their doctor". As he
says in his introduction, he doesn't know why he chose those
people.

It is a beautifully written book full of colourful and precise
observation, giving more the immediate impression of A.J. Cronin
than a Kleinian psychoanalyst. Yet the novelistic style does not
obscure a psychoanalytic mind striving to understand his
patients' lives and where possible to share his insights with
them. One is left with the impression of how crucial he was to
them and yet how little he could change their lives. Perhaps
much of general practice is accepting this paradox.

To general practitioners this book will reveal something of that
which psychoanalysis can give to their work.

To psychoanalysts it gives a fascinating insight to the "other
half", and the complexity of the problem facing the general
practitioner in disentagling the coded messages of psychosomatic
disorganisation.

Ultimately, I think psychoanalysts will be the greater
beneficiaries from this book.

                                                    Rob Hale